**Essential Trauma
and
Emergency Care**

Essential Trauma and Emergency Care

F. Wilson
V. W. Burton
A. H. Davies
A. Kilpatrick
M. B. McIllmurray
J. E. Pring

APPLETON-CENTURY-CROFTS/New York
A Division of Prentice-Hall, Inc.

Published in USA and Canada by
Appleton-Century-Crofts
A Division of Prentice-Hall, Inc.
292 Madison Avenue
New York, NY 10017

Published in UK by
MTP Press Limited
Falcon House
Lancaster, England

ISBN 0-8385-2467-2
LCCN 81-70675

Printed in Great Britain

Contents

Contributors

V. W. Burton, MB, ChB, FRCS (Ed.)
Consultant Orthopedic Surgeon,
Royal Lancaster Infirmary

A. H. Davies, MB, BS
Senior Casualty Officer,
Royal Lancaster Infirmary

A. Kilpatrick, BA, DA, LRCP, LRCS, LRFPS
Consultant Anesthetist,
Royal Lancaster Infirmary

M. B. McIllmurray, DM, MRCP
Consultant Physician,
Royal Lancaster Infirmary

J. E. Pring, MB, BS, FFARCS, DA, DRCOG, MRCS, LRCP
Senior Anesthetic Registrar,
Royal Lancaster Infirmary

F. Wilson, MB, BS, FFARCS, DA, DCH
Formerly Consultant Anesthetist,
Royal Lancaster Infirmary

Acknowledgements

We are grateful to Mr John Normanton for producing the diagrams, to Mr Philip J. Harrison, Senior Medical Photographer, Royal Lancaster Infirmary for producing the photographs, to Miss Margaret Hirst for her infinite patience and help in preparing the manuscript and to Mr David Bloomer and his staff at MTP for their guidance and encouragement at the various stages of publication.

Publisher's note

The Publishers would like to acknowledge the help of Dr Wallace Park, a colleague of Frank Wilson at the Royal Lancaster Infirmary. Following Dr Wilson's death Dr Park stepped in to assume editorial responsibility for the book and his help has been invaluable. Dr Wilson and Dr Park co-authored *Basic Resuscitation and Primary Care* published by MTP Press in 1980.

1

Function of the accident and emergency department

V. W. BURTON

Originally, Accident and Emergency departments were established to treat minor accidents and provide care for patients who were taken suddenly ill. However, recent surveys of patients attending such departments indicate that they are becoming health centres for some groups of the population. Therefore, a wide selection of patients attend these departments ranging from those suffering from minor ailments to those who have been seriously injured and who require resuscitative procedures before being admitted to hospital for definitive treatment.

Another group consists of patients who are referred for investigation by their general practitioner to the admitting surgical or medical firm on duty.

Frequently there is a delay in obtaining a bed for the patient, and medical staff may find it expedient to retain him in the Accident and Emergency department until an accurate diagnosis has been made, perhaps arranging for his direct transfer to the operating theatre if he is suffering from an acute surgical condition without prior admission to the surgical ward. The Accident and Emergency nurse is therefore involved in the management of patients suffering from a wide range of medical and surgical conditions, including trauma.

There are about 20 000 new attendances per year at the Accident and Emergency department in Lancaster. The patients are referred by their personal physicians, attend of their own accord or arrive by ambulance. Their attendance and treatment statistics are listed and discussed below.

Attendance profile at the Royal Lancaster Infirmary Accident and Emergency Department

Reason for attendance	Percentage number of patients
Non-accident	41
Sports injury	17

1

Reason for attendance	*Percentage number of patients*
Industrial or school accident	16.3
Domestic accident	13
Insect or animal involved	4
Hospital accident	2.5
Alcohol abuse	1.7
Road accident, car	1.6
Road accident, pedestrian	1.6
Road accident, motor cycle	0.7
Road accident, pedal cycle	0.6

Treatment procedures	
None	64.8
Minor surgery, including application of splint or plaster cast	14.1
Wound suturing	12.9
Removal of foreign body from eye	2.3
Removal of foreign body from elsewhere than eye	1.6
Incision and drainage of abscess	1.2
Stomach washout	0.9
Trephine and removal of nail	0.8
Removal of sutures	0.7
Resuscitative procedure	0.6
Catheterization	0.1

32% of the above patients received an injection, the most common being for anti-tetanus prophylaxis followed, in terms of frequency, by antibiotics.

37% of the patients received medication only, the most frequently prescribed being analgesics, followed by oral antibiotics.

Patients are frequently referred to the Accident and Emergency department following an injury with the request for X-ray examination. These patients are registered in the Department, examined by the Accident and Emergency doctor prior to investigation and then referred back to their general practitioner unless a fracture is identified that requires treatment.

The patients attending the Accident and Emergency department were distributed as follows

63% were discharged from hospital without follow-up being required.
11.0% were referred to their own general practitioner.
9.7% were referred to the fracture clinic following treatment.

7.4% were admitted to a local hospital.
7.3% were referred to hospitals elsewhere.

Of the remaining 1.6% some were dead on arrival, being subsequently transferred to the mortuary, while others discharged themselves from the Department.

Accident and emergency record index
The first step in patient management is the preparation of an Accident and Emergency medical record card unless there is a life-threatening condition such as an obstructed airway requiring immediate attention, or perhaps hemorrhage. During normal working hours the clerical staff at the reception desk in the department are responsible for maintaining the record index and obtaining details of all patients. The full name and address, date of birth, age, civil state, religion, occupation, general practitioner and next of kin, preferably with their telephone number are obtained and legibly recorded. Out of normal working hours the Accident and Emergency nurse is responsible for maintaining the records and recording personal details of the patients who attend.

At the Royal Lancaster Infirmary a coded system is available to record the place of incident, type of accident, arrival method and the ultimate disposal of the patient, either by discharge to his own home, with continued care from his general practitioner or admission to hospital or out-patient attendance at the Accident and Emergency department or appropriate out-patient clinic.

Computerization of notes simplifies the storage and retrieval of past records. The installation of a third generation computer, which is small and easy to use, increases the efficiency of the Accident and Emergency department and reduces the administration work load.

The efficient Accident and Emergency department can be identified from the quality of its records. The presenting complaint and all the other information contained on the record card should be legibly written by the doctor, including a brief synopsis of the accident along with the abnormal physical signs and treatment and disposal of the patient.

Nurse liaison with other hospital departments
All patients are examined by the doctor who after initial assessment may request an X-ray examination. The Accident and Emergency department should possess its own X-ray unit. Unfortunately in smaller hospitals this is not always practicable. For example in Lancaster the X-ray department is located 50 metres from the Accident and

Emergency department along a tortuous corridor. A coloured code system helps to guide strangers. Ambulant patients are asked to follow a red line 2 cm wide, painted on the corridor wall 1 metre above floor level between the two departments, thus saving the nurse time from escort duties.

Generally patients with upper limb injuries are capable of reaching the X-ray department independently, provided their damaged extremity is adequately supported in a broad arm sling. The use of metal splints is avoided because they interfere with the quality of X-ray pictures obtained.

Patients whose injuries are confined to the foot or ankle are transported in a wheelchair with the affected limb elevated on a posterior splint which may be attached to the seat of the chair. Relatives or friends are asked to accompany the patient to the X-ray department. A few words of advice on how to steer the wheelchair are helpful. Relatives are asked to pull rather than push the chair, thereby avoiding possible collision in the busy corridor, with possible further injury to the supported injured extremity.

Patients who are seriously ill or have sustained suspected pelvic, femoral or tibial fractures should be transported on a trolley (gurney), preferably with a radiolucent top so that X-ray films are obtained with a minimum amount of patient handling. A porter pushes the trolley while the nurse walks at the patient's head. She records the pulse, respiratory rate and blood pressure are recorded at regular intervals, and she alerts the doctor immediately if the patient's condition deteriorates.

The patients are asked to return to the Accident and Emergency department, bringing their X-rays with them for a further consultation with the doctor. The nurse is, therefore, constantly shepherding patients in and out of the department ensuring that no patients are lost to follow-up. Inevitably delays occur in the system, whereupon a few words of explanation to the patients and relatives will prevent a breakdown in staff–patient relationships.

The doctor, following a further interview with the patient, in conjunction with his X-rays, decides on the patient's further management. Reassurance alone may be all that is required. Alternatively the application of a splint or cast may be indicated whereas a displaced fracture or dislocation may require manipulative reduction, possibly under general anesthesia, followed by plaster cast fixation. If major surgery is required or if the domestic circumstances of the patient are unsatisfactory for home care, arrangements are made for hospital admission. The nurse is involved as a manager, informing the relatives as to the disposal of the patient. If minor surgery is indicated the patient is taken to the minor operating theatre, or to the plaster room if a fracture is present. Therefore the nurse is further involved with the deployment of patients within the department. Another of her responsibilities is to ensure that the department is adequately stocked with dressings, drugs and instruments. The rôle of the nurse is discussed more fully in chapter 2.

Frequently social problems present in the Accident and Emergency department such as when an elderly person living alone sustains a simple fracture of the wrist which requires splintage. Whereas in a younger person such a fracture presents only a minor handicap, it may be very incapacitating to the infirm patient, who lives alone, and he may need help from the social services. The nurse liaises with the medical Social Work Department based in the hospital, whose members may contact the District Social Work Department, the District Nurse and possibly also voluntary organizations who are willing to support the elderly at home with minor injuries. If adequate arrangements for the patient's welfare cannot be made immediately the patient is admitted to hospital for a day or two until support has been arranged. Management of the elderly is discussed fully in chapter 31.

2

The role of the nurse

A. H. DAVIES

When the nurse starts to work in a busy Accident and Emergency department she encounters a very different atmosphere from that existing in the wards.

All her traditional nursing virtues are necessary but the most important attribute is adaptability – a 'ready for anything, at anytime' attitude.

The type of work and work load vary from hour to hour and the nurse must be prepared to be:

(1) Occasionally bored with nothing to do.
(2) Irritated by the profusion of minor injuries and trivialities.
(3) Frightened by the sudden arrival of severely injured victims of a road traffic accident.

FRIENDLINESS

A busy department is often judged by the general atmosphere and a friendly approach is essential to patients and between colleagues be they nurses, doctors, porters, receptionists, clerical staff or cleaners. All the staff of the department need to work as a team; there is no place for rigid formality but, at the same time, discipline must be maintained and orders immediately obeyed especially in an emergency.

ROBUSTNESS AND RESILIENCE

The nurse needs to be physically strong and not easily upset by apparent chaos and confusion. She must remain undistressed by pathetic cases and tragedy, and unruffled by rudeness and abuse from difficult patients and relatives. Most nurses become used to blood and unpleasant sights but the accident patient often looks worse because he is often covered by dirt and grease with soiled and perhaps smelly clothing.

TACT

The nurse should not become exasperated, nor rebuke a stupid patient or one who is very slow, nor become visibly annoyed when faced with complaints.

The Accident and Emergency department is an 'Open House' to the general public, but however efficiently organized it is there are occasions when the smooth running is interrupted and sometimes patients are bypassed and forgotten. Most people are only conscious of their own problems and wasted time – so complaints are the natural consequence and must be dealt with sympathetically and quietly. It is always best to explain the reasons for the delays before they become too prolonged and apologize if mistakes have been made. If patients or relatives then wish to make a formal complaint they should be referred to the hospital administrator. More often they merely wish to 'let off steam' and grumble to the nurse who is naturally irritated to find that when they meet the doctor they are as pleasant and quiet as if nothing had happened.

Tact may also be required in dealing with the doctors. Through Accident and Emergency departments come a regular never ending stream of young inexperienced doctors who are often working unsupervised for the first time and who may need 'reminding' what routine treatments are available, what treatment a particular surgeon prefers, or to which clinics he may or may not refer his patients.

COOPERATION

The nurse has to deal with many officials and people other than patients.

Ambulancemen

Ambulancemen are constantly in and out of the department delivering and collecting their patients. Traditionally nursing and ambulance staff are often on first name terms and such a friendly relationship should be fostered. They are experienced and skilled and often provide valuable information regarding the history of the patient's illness, details of home conditions, the circumstances in which the patient was found, his condition when they took him into their care and his progress en route. This information often provides a baseline for future observations, may help in the diagnosis and treatment and perhaps assist the doctor to assess the prognosis.

When patients are sent home by transport the nurse should tell the ambulancemen of any special instructions which may be needed for the patient's care during the journey.

Police

The police often accompany patients to the Accident and Emergency department or arrive soon after, particularly if such cases are accident victims. They will want to know their names, addresses and next of kin, their general condition and whether the injuries are serious. They do not need detailed reports of injuries at this stage and indeed it is a breach of confidence to give them such information. The nurse, therefore, should not discuss or describe the injuries nor should she express an opinion as to whether or not the patient is intoxicated.

The police may want to interview or breathalyze the injured patient but they must not be allowed to do so without the doctor's consent. Interviews with uninjured persons or relatives is a matter of individual choice but the nurse should ask the police to conduct them away from the treatment area.

The staff of the Accident and Emergency department frequently need the help of the police, and it is in everybody's interest for all to maintain a friendly relationship. The police often contact relatives or find out what happened to personal property lost in the accident. They may retrieve the family pet and have been known to deliver false teeth and even major portions of bone left at the scene of the accident.

Another service they provide is that of escort duty if a patient has to be transferred urgently to another hospital.

The media

The nursing staff should never answer questions put to them by journalists or reporters but should refer them to a hospital administrator. It is very tempting to make a statement or give an opinion about a situation and then possibly have what one says completely distorted when it appears in print. The author once had the experience of answering the telephone when a reporter from a national newspaper rang 10 minutes after the arrival in the department of the casualties from a multiple pile-up road traffic accident. She refused to give an opinion saying 'No, I do not know how many injured there are, and we have not yet had time to sort out if anyone is really seriously hurt'. This appeared in print the next day as 'the situation in the local Accident and Emergency department was chaotic, with no-one knowing what was going on, with screaming patients and crying children left unattended'. The reporter had heard the noises of people in the background and the crying child was a patient who had nothing to do with the accident in question.

Television and film crews occasionally wish to use the Accident and Emergency department for a documentary or new feature. Again this must not be allowed without the knowledge and consent of the consultant in charge, the administrators and, not least, the patients themselves.

Relatives and friends
Relatives are often distracting in that the nurse may have to spend more time in discussing the situation with them than with the patient himself. However, relatives frequently do accompany the patient and the nurse can do much to gain their cooperation and make their stay as comfortable as possible. They should be provided with chairs to sit by the patient and shown the bell used to draw the staff's attention to any urgent need. In this way they can be useful and it saves them wandering around 'looking for someone in authority'.

If the patient is seriously ill or injured, or is being examined or treated, the relatives should be shown where to wait and the situation explained to them, and told the location of the toilets, the canteen facilities and the public telephones.

Before a seriously injured patient is seen by the relatives, they should be warned what to expect, whether he will be recognizable or whether he will be capable of recognizing his visitors. The patient and treatment area should be made clean and tidy so that blood, clothes and unpleasant-looking wounds are out of sight. The relatives should be asked to try and control themselves and not display too much emotion so they do not upset the patient and cause a deterioration in his condition. It is always wise to ask a conscious patient if he wants to see a particular relative who is asking to see him; he may not, in which case the news has to be conveyed tactfully back to the inquirer.

When the situation is stabilized a sensible relative is allowed to stay with the patient and accompany him to X-ray or to the ward. It is wise for the nurse not to discuss the patient's condition too deeply at this stage but to ask one of the more senior doctors to keep the relative informed. An incautious or erroneous prognosis from a nurse will be remembered, sometimes with bitterness, if the relative is told that the patient is going to be all right and he dies 5 minutes later.

Bereaved relatives should be provided with a place to sit and mourn, or weep if they wish. A quiet room with a closed door is more compassionate than having to express and expose their emotions in a public waiting room. The doctor may want to interview them as may the Coroner's Officer in the case of accident or sudden unexpected death. They may have to wait for other relatives to arrive, or for someone to take them home. Meanwhile the nurse should express her sympathy and be prepared to listen again to their version of the tragedy. She should provide cups of tea or coffee; occasionally sedatives may be suggested if the relatives are distraught or hysterical but before these are administered, the nurse should ask whether the patient is already taking medication. However, some authorities do not approve of sedation and many psychiatrists believe that generally a conscious and unsedated period is necessary for the ultimate acceptance of bereavement, so that the handing out of diazepam all round is inadvisable.

Before the relatives leave the department the nurse must inform the family doctor of the situation because later on he may be called out to treat them in their home.

Belligerent, noisy or disruptive relatives and friends must be handled tactfully. This problem is dealt with in the section on violence (p. 289).

Organization of the Accident and Emergency department

The organization and smooth running of the department, the deployment of staff and decisions regarding facilities and equipment should be agreed in cooperation with the medical staff.

PATIENT FLOW

Special signposted areas close to the examination and treatment rooms should be allocated for the patient awaiting the initial examination by the doctor, X-ray examination or after radiography. Patients are then less likely to be missed or bypassed. Similarly, the patient's notes should be placed in special places so that the nurses and doctors can see instantly how many are waiting at any stage of management.

NURSE LOCATION

In an ideal situation there are two nurses for every patient/doctor consultation, so that one stays with the patient to carry out any observations and treatment ordered while the other acts as a runner to acquire any equipment which might be needed.

CHAPERONAGE

When a female patient is being examined, in a closed off area by a male doctor, it may be necessary for a chaperone to be present to avoid allegations of assault or indecency. It is perhaps surprising that such complaints do not necessarily come from young and attractive patients; often the accusation comes from the most unexpected source. Therefore, if a doctor asks a nurse to remain in the room while he examines a female patient she should do so. Occasionally of course the reverse is true – and as a female doctor the author has occasionally been reluctant to examine a male patient by herself.

DECISIONS
Which nurse is to perform what duties must rest with the sister or nursing officer in charge*. When a new nurse arrives in the department she is shown where everything is stored and allowed to work with a more experienced nurse until she is familiar with the layout and the nursing procedures. She should not be afraid to ask for guidance from a more experienced colleague if her instructions are not clear or if she has not carried out a particular procedure before.

DEPLOYMENT OF STAFF
The work load is unpredictable from one hour to the next and consequently the staff may be very busy or have little to do. Advantage of the slack periods must be taken and activities other than patient care performed when circumstances permit. They are delegated by the nurse in charge:

(1) Cleaning and tidying the department.
(2) Making use of relevant books, cassettes and video cassettes.
(3) Organizing projects for junior nurse participation.
(4) Conducting and participating in continuing education.

STAFF ROTATION
A deployment chart or board enables nurses to rotate and share the various activities, thus obtaining experience in all areas of the department. Furthermore it discloses the location of the staff when they are urgently needed.

PATIENT LOCATION
A similar board is useful for patient details, particularly stretcher cases, such as their time of arrival and for whom or what they are waiting. It ensures that patients are not forgotten or left lying around without supervision, observation or regular review.

*In the UK a sister is a fully qualified state registered nurse of senior rank. 'Sister' does not imply that she belongs to a particular religious denomination.

3

Wounds

V. W. BURTON

Causes

In Lancaster 13% of the patients attending the Accident and Emergency department do so for the treatment of wounds. Although most wounds result from domestic accidents, involving knives, tin cans or broken glass, they are also inflicted by needles, lead pencils, thorns, rusty nails and gardening implements. The fingers are most commonly injured at home, the face and scalp in road traffic accidents, whereas limb wounds frequently follow sport injuries. Industrial machinery and vehicles are responsible for many of the wounds that present as a combination of lacerations and crush injuries.

Types

Wounds may be classified according to their appearance as incised, lacerated or punctured. They require appropriate treatment to ensure rapid healing with the minimum of complications. All wounds are contaminated and are, therefore, potentially infected. Consequently wound management is based on the principles of removing contamination and providing skin cover, thus protecting the wound from further bacterial infection.

Treatment of wounds

CLINICAL HISTORY

The clinical history, time, place and mode of wounding are recorded. These are important because the wound sustained by contact with a muddy football boot on the football pitch requires a different approach from one inflicted by a clean razor blade. The history of a penetrating wound, particularly if due to broken glass, often indicates the possible retention of foreign material. X-rays may then confirm the diagnosis, as 90% of glass used in the United Kingdom is radio-opaque. The nurse is usually the first member of the medical team to interview the patient and in the absence of the doctor she may decide to alert the X-ray department.

12

EXAMINATION OF WOUNDS

Examination of the wound should be carried out under adequate illumination. If the wound is trivial the patient may remain seated, otherwise he should lie down. Any temporary dressings applied prior to the patient attending the hospital are retained as they may provide a rough estimation of blood loss.

The initial inspection of the wound determines its size, site and degree of contamination. The site of the wound may indicate to the medical or nursing staff the possibility of injury to underlying nerves or tendons.

Peripheral nerves carry sensory fibres for sensation, and motor fibres for voluntary movements. Division of such a nerve results in the loss of tactile sensation and joint position sense and also of the specific voluntary movement activated by those muscles previously supplied by the peripheral nerve. Peripheral nerve function is always assessed before treating wounds of an extremity. The extent of sensory loss is decided by testing for sensibility to light touch and pin prick. Complete paralysis of the muscle whose nerve supply has been interrupted may be demonstrated by asking the patient to perform a specific movement, observing the extremity closely and noting the absence of any movement, and also by palpating the muscle and noticing the absence of contraction. Care is necessary in deciding whether any movement present is actually normal. Sometimes other muscles, unaffected by the nerve damage, try to compensate and produce movement which is almost similar to that produced by the paralysed muscle.

A knowledge of anatomy is required to make a diagnosis. Complete division of the median nerve at the wrist results in altered sensibility over the anterior aspect of the thumb, index, long finger and a portion of the ring finger in addition to paralysis of the muscles situated over the ball of the thumb. Complete division of the radial nerve in the arm results in impaired sensibility over the dorsum of the thumb and paralysis of the muscles which extend the wrist. Complete division of the ulnar nerve at the wrist results in numbness of the little finger and half of the ring finger with paralysis of the small muscles in the hand apart from those in the fleshy portion of the thumb.

The division of a tendon should also be suspected with palmar or digital wounds where loss of voluntary movement is demonstrated. Suspected tendon or nerve damage in a limb injury calls for admission of the patient and exploration of the wound under general anesthesia, which provides ideal operating conditions, including the use of an exsanguinating tourniquet to obtain a completely bloodless field.

Use of camera

If a Polaroid camera is available the wound is photographed and the print kept as a record of the state of the wound on admission. It is then available to all medical and nursing staff, obviating the need for repeated removal of the dressing with the possible recurrence of hemorrhage and introduction of infection.

If blood loss has been considerable, or there are signs and symptoms of surgical shock, a sample of blood is taken by venepuncture and sent to the laboratory for grouping and cross-matching. An intravenous infusion is started forthwith.

Removal of clothing

Once the hemorrhage is controlled the patient is examined in more detail. Clothing must be removed, if necessary by cutting along the seams. Where one arm is injured, the shirt or blouse is easily removed if the normal arm is withdrawn from the clothing first and then the garment pulled over the patient's head.

Most difficulty is encountered with motor cycle victims especially when removing footwear where a crush injury of the extremity is suspected. Two nurses are required, one to steady the limb while the other completely unties or cuts the laces and slowly removes the boot or shoe. The pain caused by these manoeuvres may be reduced by the administration 50% nitrous oxide in oxygen by face mask. The patient is asked to take six deep breaths over a 40 second period to ensure the concentration of nitrous oxide in the blood is sufficient to produce the necessary degree of analgesia.

Rings should be removed immediately from damaged fingers to prevent further swelling which may make later removal impossible. If removing the ring proves difficult and the skin is not lacerated the application of soap with immersion of the hand in cold water and gentle easing of the ring over the proximal interphalangeal joint will usually be successful. The only alternative is to divide the ring with a small circular saw but the patient's permission must always be sought prior to this manoeuvre and it should only be contemplated if the circulation of the finger is in jeopardy.

NURSE HAND CARE AND 'SCRUBBING UP'

Work in the Accident and Emergency department involves frequent handling of dirty clothes, dirty patients and dirty purulent and bloody wounds. If cross-infection is to be avoided, ideally the doctor and the nurse should clean and disinfect their hands between each patient contact. This is usually impracticable and often downright impossible as for example when a serious emergency is suddenly brought in while the nurse is in the middle of treating another less urgent patient. Practicality, therefore, demands that the nurse should keep her hands *reasonably* clean all the time and specially clean for some maneuver.

The nurse should aim to keep her hands 'socially' clean, scrubbing them for 1 – 2 minutes removing visible dirt and debris from the nails which should be kept short and neatly trimmed. She should use an antiseptic soap until the hands look clean, followed by an antiseptic 'scrubbing' lotion, e.g. one containing compound iodine or chlorhexidine. Similar spirit based 'hand rubs' are available which do not require water for their effective use, and these may be used between treating patients provided the hands have not been grossly contaminated. The hands should be dried after every water cleansing because the skin becomes excoriated and organisms are more likely to survive on a moist warm surface. Paper towels are satisfactory for ordinary use, or sterile paper towels if the procedure demands a sterile technique such as those involving open wounds. Hot air hand dryers are a useful adjunct but tend to be time consuming.

When the nurse is actually involved in dressing or suturing a wound or assisting a minor operation she should wear sterile gloves. The alternative is the combination of clean hands and a scrupulous no-touch technique. This technique of never touching the wound with the hands but always employing sterile forceps for holding swabs and applying dressings is probably the best safeguard against cross-infection in such an unsterile place as the Accident and Emergency department.

At the end of the day or period of duty most nurses' hands need hand cream to restore the natural oils that have been washed away. A jar of soft and pleasant-smelling hand cream should be kept in the nurses toilet or staff room to help her hands healthy and presentable and make her feel less conscious of her distinctive 'hospital smell' when she returns home.

SKIN CLOSURE
The majority of wounds treated in the Accident and Emergency department are situated on the hand, the face and the distal portion of the extremities. Minor wounds are treated in the examination cubicle while more extensive wounds are treated in the theatre.

If a central sterile supply department exists within the hospital, packs containing suture materials, double wrapped in sterile paper towels, are available in addition to supplementary packs containing sterile towels to drape around the wound.

The first procedure for the nurse is the preparation of the trolley (cart). A paper mask is donned prior to washing her hands and drying them with a clean paper towel. The top of the trolley is cleaned with soap and water and a paper towel and is then allowed to dry following the application of surgical spirit. On the bottom shelf of the trolley the nurse places the 'non-sterile' items such as adhesive plaster dressings, bottles of an antiseptic lotion, a local analgesic solution, scissors, syringes and needles in addition to a pack of sterile rubber gloves of appropriate size for the doctor.

The trolley is then moved to the treatment area where the doctor, with the assistance of the nurse, will examine, clean and close the wound.

Wound preparation

The nurse cleans the area around the wound using an antiseptic solution such as Savlon, which is a combination of chlorhexidine and cetrimide in an aqueous solution, or Betadine. The solution is emptied into a small bowl containing cotton wool balls which are grasped in sterile forceps, used to clean the skin and then discarded into a different container.

In areas such as the scalp, scissors are used to remove hair for a distance of 2 cm around the laceration while a small razor is more appropriate for skin wounds on the extremities.

The use of adhesive sutures

Minor wounds, especially those on the face, may be treated successfully by closure with adhesive sutures. This technique is especially useful for clean, incised wounds which must be thoroughly cleansed prior to skin closure. To achieve success the doctor and nurse must work together as a team. The skin around the wound must be dry and free of hair for a distance of at least 2 cm on all sides. The application of ether to 'de-fat' the skin is not necessary. The sutures are applied by the nurse at right angles to the wound while the doctor approximates the wound margins. Therefore, they are applied under slight tension, and are arranged at about 0.5 cm intervals over the length of the wound. Sterile swabs are used to absorb any blood which may ooze on to the skin surface. 'Plastic skin' obtained from an aerosol can be applied over the surface of the wound and sutures, taking care to protect the patient's eyes.

CLOSURE OF MORE EXTENSIVE WOUNDS

The wound is irrigated with normal saline and cleaned with Savlodil or Betadine to enable the doctor to decide whether general anaesthesia or local analgesia is appropriate.

General anaesthesia is preferable where an extensive abraded wound is complicated by diffuse contamination with dirt which if not removed results in the formation of a permanent tattoo. If a general anaesthetic is necessary the patient is moved to the minor surgical theatre where the nurse provides a trolley for wound closure including a sterile brush which is helpful in removing extensive contamination. However, most wounds in the Accident and Emergency department are managed under local analgesia (chapter 13) or without analgesia. If the wound is small and there is no suggestion of retained foreign material, the minor discomfort associated with the insertion of two sutures, using a sharp atraumatic needle, is no greater than the injection required to introduce the local analgesic.

Use of local analgesia

A popular local analgesic is 1% lignocaine (lidocaine) without adrenalin (epinephrine p. 127). Lignocaine is available in ampoules, in a multidose container or in a cartridge syringe used in dental practice. The masked doctor, after washing his arms and forearms thoroughly, puts on sterile gloves and accepts the sterile 10 ml syringe from the nurse, after she has split the seal on its protective package. A 19 gauge (G) needle is then attached to the syringe and the rubber diaphragm of the multidose vial is cleaned with spirit. The vial is held inverted prior to puncture of the diaphragm and subsequent aspiration of the local analgesic solution into the syringe.

For infiltration of the solution the needle is changed to either a 23 or a finer 25 gauge (G). The 25 G needle is preferable especially when performing a digital nerve block, as penetration of the skin in the palm of the hand or sole of the foot is particularly painful. Between 1 and 10 ml of 1% lignocaine are usually sufficient for most wounds. Introduction of the needle and infiltration under the wound edge is a satisfactory technique and is described on p. 110.

Wounds of the fingers are most easily sutured under local analgesia achieved by a ring block. With this technique 1% lignocaine is injected at the base of the finger and deposited around the site of the digital nerve. 3 ml of the 1% lignocaine solution without adrenalin are injected on both sides of the base of the finger, the needle being inserted posteriorly where the skin is thinner; infiltration is completed slightly anterior to the proximal phalanx. A further infiltration of 2 ml over the dorsum of the finger achieves the required analgesia. After the injection of the local analgesic at least 10 min should elapse before any surgical procedure is commenced, permitting adequate time for the lignocaine solution to produce its analgesic effect.

The efficiency of the infiltration is tested by estimating the response to pin prick, using a sterile needle in the vicinity of the wound.

Wound preparation

The wound is again cleaned thoroughly with an antiseptic solution and should deeper exploration of the wound reveal further contamination, irrigation with sterile normal saline is helpful. If the wound is extensive this is achieved by pouring the solution from a sterile container into the wound or alternatively, a 50 ml syringe containing saline for the irrigation of smaller wounds.

Suture technique

When the doctor is satisfied that all obvious contamination has been removed, suturing may commence. The nurse removes the outer layer of the suture pack enclosing sterile towels, disposable containers and swabs, needle holder, artery forceps, dissecting forceps, suture scissors and a small scalpel handle with number 11 and number 15 scalpel blades.

Sterile towels are arranged round the wound to avoid possible contamination from the surrounding area. The doctor removes any devitalized tissue and after wound excision is complete he asks the nurse for suitable suture material. For general purpose use a 3/0 Dexon or a 3/0 black silk suture on an atraumatic 25 mm taper cut needle is satisfactory. For facial lacerations a 20 mm deeper cutting needle is used with either 5/0 Dexon, black silk or a synthetic non-absorbable suture such as Proline.

Interrupted sutures are inserted with the nurse acting as the assistant. She simultaneously reassures the patient and encourages him to keep still. She trims the sutures leaving ends of about 5 mm in length for their easy removal. Apart from cutting the sutures she also maintains a supply of further suture material and frequently swabs the wound, using a pair of dissecting forceps to handle the sterile swabs which she drops after use into a container on the non-sterile portion of the trolley.

Suture removal

Sutures are removed from facial lacerations after 5 days but sutures in the extremities should remain for 10 days. Fine Dexon sutures used for skin lacerations and in children or to close wounds subsequently covered by a plaster of Paris cast may be left indefinitely as they are biodegradable (dissolved by the body) and disappear after 6 weeks.

Dressings

After being sutured the wound is either left exposed or covered by a dressing. Facial and scalp lacerations are better treated by exposure because dressings are difficult to keep in place in hairy regions. Consequently 'plastic skin' from an aerosol is used to seal the wound, but care must be taken to protect the patient's eyes and mucous membranes during its application.

In the extremities a non-adhesive, dry, absorbent dressing, held in position either by an elastic adhesive bandage or by a cotton conforming bandage, improve the patient's comfort. With finger injuries a satisfactory alternative is the use of tube gauze whereby a cylinder of gauze is applied to the finger giving a dressing of three or four layers thick. Care is taken when using the applicator that no tension exists around the base of the finger to compromise the circulation. Dressings on areas such as the chest wall or axilla are supported by a large pad held in position by Netelast.

Splintage

A broad arm sling is advisable for wounds distal to the elbow. The patient is instructed to keep his hand elevated to minimize post-operative swelling, especially for wounds of the fingers or hand. He is told to regularly flex and extend the fingers and wrists as early mobility with hand injuries prevents the possible accumulation of protein-rich fluid within the tissues which can organize into fibrous tissue and cause permanent joint stiffness. He is further instructed to maintain shoulder movements by placing his hand alternately behind the back of his head and behind the small of his back at least once every 2 hours to avoid the development of shoulder stiffness.

Wounds of the sole of the foot are protected by bulky dressings and the patient is advised to keep his foot elevated as much as possible and to maintain movements at the ankle. For mobility he is provided with crutches and advised on their use.

Types of wounds

Heavily contaminated wounds such as those resulting from dog bites should not be sutured. They should be completely cleaned and if necessary the wound should be extended to permit further irrigation of the depths of the wound. No attempt is made to suture the wound which is left open and is covered by a non-stick dressing. If possible the damaged area should be rested in an elevated position and prophylactic

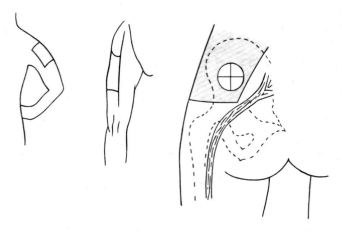

Figure 3.1   Sites for intramuscular injection

antibiotics administered. Provided there is no history of penicillin sensitivity, 500 mg of Magnapen (a combination of flucloxacillin 250 mg and ampicillin 250 mg) is injected into the deep muscles over the upper outer quadrant of the buttock (Figure 3.1). The patient then receives 500 mg of Magnapen 6 hourly by mouth for a 5 day period.

Small wounds resulting from high pressure injection of paint or grease may appear insignificant but they are notorious for causing permanent disability. These injuries are best treated by immediate admission to a specialized unit.

Fish hooks may transfix the ear lobe or become firmly embedded in the face or hand. They may be extracted by administering local analgesia in a 1% lignocaine solution manipulating the shank of the hook to complete its penetration of the skin so that the projecting barb can be removed using a small wire cutter. Once the barb has been removed the rest of the hook is readily removed from the soft tissues. Complete excision of the area is advisable in view of the risk of infection.

FOREIGN BODIES

A patient may attend complaining of a painful lump with a history of a related penetrating injury received several weeks previously, possibly from a lead pencil or thorn. The lump, known as a foreign body granuloma, is due to the development of a surrounding fibrous coat around the retained foreign material. Treatment is by excision, usually under local analgesia. The nurse prepares a trolley using a similar technique to that used for wound sutures.

Patients with retained foreign matter, such as air gun pellets or needles, who present immediately after injury are best treated in the main operating theatre under general anaesthesia unless the objects are readily obvious on wound inspection.

BURNS

Burns are caused by dry heat whereas scalds are due to moist heat. The diagnosis of a burn is obvious with local charring or blistering of the skin. Minor burns are treated on an out-patient basis in the Accident and Emergency department while those patients who have extensive burns in excess of 10% of the body surface require resuscitation with intravenous fluids to compensate for the loss of plasma from the circulation.

On reception of such a patient and after consultation with the doctor, the nurse prepares a trolley for an intravenous infusion and arranges for admission to a specialized burns unit.

Pain relief

The patient is generally in a state of severe distress and the first step in his management should be pain relief. In the adult 10 mg intravenous morphine sulphate is given and repeated if necessary. Intramuscular morphine is avoided because of poor tissue perfusion secondary to hypovolemic shock which prevents absorption until the circulation has returned to normal.

Extent

The extent of the burn is assessed by 'The Rule of Nine'. Each arm represents 9% of the body surface, each leg 18%, the front of the chest and abdomen 18%, the back of the chest and abdomen 18%, head and neck 9% and the external genitalia 1%.

Depth

After determining the extent of the burn, an assessment of the depth is important. In a deep wound all layers of the skin are destroyed, whereas in a superficial burn of the skin elements such as the hair follicles remain. The differentiation between deep and superficial can be difficult but a deep burn usually presents a charred appearance with complete anaesthesia of the area. The superficial burn has a blistered appearance with underlying oedematous damaged epithelium which is very sensitive.

The differentiation between the two is important as a deep burn heals after separation of the eschar (dead skin). Consequently healing is prolonged and may only be achieved by split skin grafting, whereas a superficial burn heals rapidly provided that infection does not supervene.

The aim of treatment is to cover the skin as soon as possible in an attempt to prevent infection, reduce scarring and to thereby maintain function.

Local treatment

After the doctor has assessed the burn, the nurse is asked to dress the damaged area. She adopts a sterile technique wearing a mask and sterile gloves after a full surgical hand scrub. The adjacent areas are screened by sterile towels. The burned area is gently cleaned with antiseptic solution and any necrotic skin, foreign material, and adherent clothing, are removed. Blisters are trimmed, using sterile scissors.

A sterile non-stick dressing, such as Melolin, or alternatively vaseline gauze, is applied if the burn is situated on an extremity while burns on the face may be treated by exposure with topical application of an antibiotic powder such as Polybactrin (neomycin, polymyxin and bacitracin).

If contiguous surfaces of adjacent fingers are involved, care must be taken to ensure that the burned surfaces are kept apart by an intervening dressing. The affected part is elevated and the patient instructed how to perform suitable exercises to prevent joint stiffness and the possible development of later scar contracture.

Dressings are changed at 3–4 day intervals, always under aseptic conditions. If the burn is deep a thick eschar develops and the periphery of this is trimmed with sterile scissors at each dressing to encourage skin healing. Should the eschar be greater than 2.5 cm square it is best excised followed immediately, if there is no infection, by the application of a split skin graft.

If infection develops in a deep burn, pus forms around the edges of the eschar and the nurse obtains a sample of the discharge for bacteriological investigation prior to dressing the wound. Once infection has become established, regular daily dressings are necessary, with suitable oral or intramuscular antibiotics indicated by the sensitivity as reports on the organisms isolated from the specimen of pus sent for culture.

Local applications of ointment, such as Aserbine or Malatex (both contain, in different proportions, propylene glycol, malic acid, benzoic acid and salicylic acid and will accelerate separation of the slough leaving a clean, granulating surface suitable for the application of a split skin graft).

Superficial burns, provided infection does not supervene, heal rapidly but the nurse must be ever vigilant and report any evidence of infection present when dressing the wound to the doctor.

Electric burns require special care because inevitably deep tissues are irreversibly damaged. Early excision of the necrotic tissue is the treatment of choice followed by early grafting.

Chemical burns most frequently encountered are those due to sulphuric acid leaking from batteries or are caused by caustic soda. If the patient attends immediately after contact, the most effective first aid measure is immersion of the affected area in water to dilute the acid or alkali. Thereafter, management of the burn is similar to that of a thermal injury depending on whether the resultant skin damage is deep or superficial.

Scalds, frequently encountered in domestic accidents due to boiling water or steam, are treated in the same manner as burns.

Wound complications
HEMORRHAGE
The most serious immediate complication of a wound is hemorrhage which may be capillary, venous or arterial.

Capillary hemorrhage

In capillary hemorrhage there is a steady oozing from the small vessels in the wound margins which often seal themselves off by the time the patient reaches hospital. However if bleeding persists capillary hemorrhage is easily controlled by exerting local pressure over a sterile pad. In fact, this is true of most cases of troublesome hemorrhage encountered in the Accident and Emergency department, and packs of sterile pads are therefore kept readily available for this purpose in all the examination areas.

Venous hemorrhage

In venous hemorrhage, for example from ruptured varicose veins in the lower leg, there is a steady oozing of dark blood from both ends of the damaged vessel. The blood does not spurt out so that local pressure and preferably elevation of the injured part, followed by application of a sterile dressing and support with a crepe bandage are sufficient to stop the bleeding. If a varicose vein at the ankle is the site of hemorrhage the patient should lie down with the foot elevated on a small stool. Elevation should be maintained for about 15 min to ensure clotting in the thin walled vessel before allowing the patient to stand.

Arterial hemorrhage

Arterial hemorrhage is more dramatic and is readily diagnosed because blood spurts out under arterial pressure. If severe blood loss occurs before the patient reaches hospital due to rupture of a major blood vessel, hypovolemic shock (p. 139) may be established, accompanied by its typical clinical signs, so that the patient appears anxious, the skin is cold and clammy to the touch, respiration rate is shallow and rapid, the pulse is rapid and the blood pressure is low. The nurse should always remember these signs when receiving an accident victim, especially if the appearance of the clothing suggests a severe arterial hemorrhage. Wounds of the scalp in particular bleed profusely and blood loss may be considerable because of the rich anastomoses between arteries residing in the scalp tissues. Consequently, a patient waiting in the department with scalp lacerations may continue to bleed and the nurse should ensure that they are never left unobserved.

Indiscriminate attempts to locate ruptured arteries with forceps in a contaminated wound are unwise, especially in the unconscious patient. This practice, which is seldom effective, can result in tissue damage and certainly results in dissemination of bacteria within the wound. First aid treatment of arterial hemorrhage is to apply a sterile dressing and exert local pressure. If profuse arterial bleeding persists, a tourniquet may be applied to the padded limb proximal to the wound. A pneumatic tourniquet inflated to about 250 mmHg is preferable, but it should not remain inflated for longer than 1 hour.

TETANUS
Organism
Even when a wound or burn is treated by closure or dressings, there is a definite risk of significant infection developing and none is more serious than tetanus. Tetanus may develop in association with any type of wound but puncture wounds contaminated with soil are particularly liable. The bacteria responsible are called *Clostridium tetani* which only grow and multiply in conditions of poor oxygenation. Acute tetanus develops within 2 weeks of infection. Initially the patient is restless followed within a day or two with severe muscle spasms. The mortality is considerable and prophylaxis is therefore of paramount importance.

Prophylactic antibiotics
Thorough cleansing of the wound and excision of all dead tissue are routinely performed as is the administration of one vial of Triplopen by deep intramuscular injection provided there is no history of penicillin sensitivity. Triplopen is a combination of three different penicillins which ensures an adequate blood level of antibiotic for 3 days. If wound contamination is severe, either the intramuscular Triplopen is repeated after 3 days or the patient is started immediately on a 10 day course of 250 mg flucloxacillin 6 hourly by mouth.

Immunization
Most people, especially agricultural workers and gardeners, should be immunized against tetanus. If not previously immunized, active immunization is achieved by stimulating the production of antibodies by the injection of an antigen. The antigen used for active tetanus immunization is tetanus toxoid (available in the United Kingdom as adsorbed tetanus vaccine) which is relatively non-toxic but when injected produces an antibody response. Three subcutaneous injections of 0.5 ml tetanus toxoid at intervals of 8 weeks and 6 months produces an adequate antibody response. A repeat 'booster' subcutaneous injection of 0.5 ml tetanus toxoid should be administered every 4 years.

The patient usually knows if he has been adequately immunized against tetanus, and the nurse should enter such information in the case notes. If there is any doubt he should be regarded as being inadequately immunized and the prophylactic immunization schedule started as soon as possible after injury.

If previously immunized, active immunization was conferred by the appropriate number of tetanus toxoid injections. Treatment now consists of intramuscular penicillin and a booster subcutaneous injection of 0.5 ml of tetanus toxoid. Alternatively, the tetanus toxoid and penicillin can be mixed in the same syringe and given by intramuscular injection.

The patient who has never previously received tetanus toxoid or who has only received one dose of tetanus toxoid is susceptible to the disease and should be protected by the administration of human tetanus immunoglobulin. Human tetanus immunoglobulin, BP is available in vials containing 250 international units of tetanus anti-toxin in 1 ml of solution. This anti-toxin provides passive immunization against tetanus but the immunity conferred is only temporary. Tetanus anti-toxin 1 ml subcutaneously is administered in conjunction with tetanus toxoid 0.5 ml subcutaneously as soon as possible after the tetanus-susceptible patient has sustained the wound.

Human tetanus immunoglobulin and tetanus toxoid should be administered with separate syringes and into separate sites because tetanus toxoid in simple solution is unsuitable for concurrent administration with human tetanus immunoglobulin. The dose of human tetanus immunoglobulin for children is the same as that for adults; it should never be given intravenously.

The administration of human tetanus anti-toxin does not obviate the need for debridement, wound toilet or the use of antibiotics.

If more than 24 hours have elapsed since the wound was sustained or if there is a risk of heavy contamination with *Clostridium tetani*, 2 ml (500 international units) of human tetanus immunoglobulin should be given subcutaneously, irrespective of whether or not the patient has been immunized before.

Follow-up treatment

Before the patient leaves the Accident and Emergency department, arrangements are made for his follow-up, either at the department or the office of his family physician. His progress is checked, usually after 24 hours, to ensure that the dressing does not require changing and that local swelling has not compromised the circulation. The patient is asked to contact the hospital if he develops local pain, if any discharge appears through the dressing, or if any new symptoms develop that are attributable to the injury.

4

Abdominal emergencies

V. W. BURTON

The average district general hospital in the United Kingdom admits 7000 patients annually suffering from acute abdominal pain. The pattern of hospital admissions has changed in our larger cities over the past 12 years due in part to an increasingly mobile population. Many patients arrive initially with abdominal pain for examination at the Accident and Emergency department whereas others are admitted direct to the medical or surgical ward after communication by telephone between their general practitioner and hospital staff.

The presenting symptoms include acute abdominal pain with vomiting. If the patient is dehydrated due to prolonged vomiting or is suffering from gastrointestinal hemorrhage he will require intravenous fluids and a specimen of blood taken for cross-matching, full blood count, packed cell volume and electrolyte estimation. Vomitus may be brown and smell fecal in intestinal obstruction while in vomitus associated with gastric hemorrhage the contained blood resembles coffee grounds or appears as frank red blood if hemorrhage is brisk and recent.

Examination frequently reveals evidence of peritoneal irritation with tenderness and possibly abdominal distension. The patient may feel warm and perspire due to infection.

Aetiology

The commonest surgical causes of the acute abdominal syndrome in order of frequency are:

Appendicitis
Renal or biliary colic
Acute intestinal obstruction
Diverticulitis of the large bowel
Pelvic inflammatory disease and conditions of the female genital tract, such as ectopic gestation or a ruptured or twisted ovarian cyst
Perforation of peptic ulcer or large bowel
Intraperitoneal hemorrhage

26

Apart from surgical causes of the acute abdominal syndrome there are other conditions of a medical nature, such as gastroenteritis due to either chemical or bacteriological food poisoning that can present with similar signs and symptoms. Other examples are pneumonia especially in young children, pleurisy and shingles, all of which can produce symptoms and signs referred to the abdomen.

INJURY

Trauma is an infrequent cause of the acute abdominal syndrome but an intra-abdominal injury should always be considered when a victim with multiple injuries is assessed in the Accident and Emergency department. The abdominal contents may be injured either by blunt trauma, as caused by a seat belt restraining an accident victim at the time of impact, or by a penetrating wound, possibly inflicted by a knife or piece of glass. It is quite possible for penetrating wounds located in the chest or pelvis to involve the abdominal viscera, and if a history of wounding with a lengthy implement is obtained or suspected no attempt should be made to suture such a wound in the Accident and Emergency department. The appropriate management is the immediate admission of the patient with subsequent exploration of the wound in the operating theatre so that a formal laparotomy may be undertaken in case the wound extends to the peritoneal cavity. The author has seen a youth, 18 years of age, walk into the hospital with a piece of glass sticking out posteriorly from his upper chest. At exploration the glass was found to be stiletto-like in shape and had passed through his left lung, diaphragm, left kidney and intestine.

Abdominal trauma may produce bleeding due to division of a major artery or laceration of a vascular organ such as the spleen or liver. The spleen is the most frequently injured abdominal organ because it is particularly friable, has a long pedicle and lies in relation to the 9th, 10th and 11th ribs. Rupture of the spleen may occasionally be due to open injury but the most frequent cause is blunt trauma to the left lower hemithorax. It usually produces a hemoperitoneum (blood in the peritoneal cavity). Intraperitoneal hemorrhage presents as an acute abdomen with local pain and tenderness accompanied by signs of hypovolemic shock (p. 139).

PERFORATIONS

Damage to the gastrointestinal tract causing perforation allows escape of intestinal contents into the peritoneal cavity and produces the abdominal pain of early peritonitis. Pancreatic rupture releases secretions rich in enzymes which produce fat necrosis within the peritoneal cavity.

Symptoms

The patient feels nauseated, vomits, looks ill and the features of hypo-volemic shock are evident (p. 139). Abdominal pain is severe and may radiate to the back and shoulders. Radiation of pain to the shoulder regions is common when the peritoneum lining the diaphragm is irritated because the phrenic nerves supplying the diaphragm arise from the mid-cervical region. Rupture of the stomach and/or duodenum permits the escape of hydrochloric acid, enzymes and partially digested food into the peritoneal cavity, while large bowel rupture results in a faecal peritonitis. All these initially produce severe pain and tenderness of the abdomen. The patient tends to remain still, does not like to be moved and breathes shallowly.

The nurse, being the first professional member of the Accident and Emergency team to contact the patient with abdominal symptoms, is in a unique position to obtain useful information as to the mode of onset of his present illness and of its subsequent development. She determines if there is a precipitating factor, such as injury, or whether he has been admitted to the hospital before with a similar condition. Relatives, witnesses or friends are questioned regarding the patient's illness, particularly if he is shocked, very deaf or otherwise incapable of providing an adequate history. The nurse enquires whether any one else who has been in close contact with the patient has experienced similar symptoms, particularly abdominal pain, vomiting or diarrhea, which together suggest the presence of an infective condition such as gastro-enteritis.

Patient management

The patient with abdominal pain is placed on a moveable trolley (gurney) to facilitate further investigation by the medical staff.

The nurse then records the temperature, pulse rate, respiratory rate and blood pressure on the front of the emergency card and also on a separate sheet which is later filed with the in-patient notes.

The oral temperature recorded under the tongue is the most accurate. However, the axillary recording avoids the risk of thermometer breakage if the patient is confused, unconscious or epileptic. The rectal temperature is readily obtained in children under 1 year of age.

The pulse rate may be counted by palpation of the radial artery at the wrist but if the patient is shocked the radial pulse may be feeble and difficult to feel. Under these circumstances the femoral pulse may be palpated at the groin, midway between the pubic tubercle and the anterior margin of the iliac crest. As an alternative the pulse rate may be obtained by auscultation of the heart.

The blood pressure is obtained using a sphygmomanometer with the cuff applied to the arm midway between the shoulder and the elbow. If the patient is seriously ill and recordings of the pulse and blood pressure are required every 10 minutes, it is convenient to leave the cuff in position ensuring that it is always completely deflated after taking every blood pressure reading.

The nurse reassures the patient as every procedure is started, adopting an optimistic attitude towards the illness. She then assists the doctor who assesses the patient by obtaining a full history, performing a general examination and paying special attention to palpation and auscultation of the abdomen. The nurse is frequently able to augment the history with her knowledge of the patient's condition since his admission to the unit. She requests any previous medical records of the patient's previous illnesses and treatment from the medical records officer.

OTHER DUTIES

Personal belongings are placed in a plastic bag, secured to the trolley base. The patient is then wheeled into the cubicle where his outer garments are removed and stored in another plastic bag which also remains on the trolley, clearly marked with his name, address and emergency number. Dentures are removed and stored likewise in a clearly marked container which remains with his other belongings.

A vomit bowl and packet of paper tissues (wipes) are kept close by and any vomitus is retained for inspection. If vomiting is severe the patient is usually more comfortable lying on his side. Mucus and vomitus retained in the mouth are removed by tissues or by means of suction. If the patient is then able to carry out his own oral toilet, he is provided with a tray containing a small bowl of water, a tumbler of water for washing out his mouth, a container and paper towels. He is told not to drink or eat because a general anesthetic may be required later, and because any peritoneal soiling present will increase if there is a major perforation in the upper gastrointestinal tract.

Auscultation of the abdomen and chest is important, perhaps revealing the absence of bowel sounds suggestive of peritonitis or signs indicative of pleurisy or pneumonia. In a 'traumatic acute abdomen' the finding of bowel sounds in the chest suggest rupture of the diaphragm.

Distension of the abdomen frequently develops in patients who present with an acute abdomen following trauma. This may be due to inefficient peristaltic action of the bowel, paralytic ileus or intra-peritoneal hemorrhage. Frequent measurements of the abdominal circumference at the level of the umbilicus is useful in the monitoring of the patient's progress while he remains in the department.

A rectal examination is helpful in the diagnosis of abdominal disease, it is less helpful in the diagnosis of intra-abdominal trauma but it should be performed in most cases. An examination tray is prepared containing large and medium size disposable gloves, lubricating jelly, small dressing packs and a paper bag for soiled swabs. The patient is informed about the examination and asked to empty his bladder if possible. Privacy for the patient must be assured. The male patient usually manages to micturate into a urinal but if he has difficulty in passing urine while supine, he is allowed to stand provided there is no clinical evidence of shock. The female patient sometimes may find difficulty in using a bedpan balanced on top of a trolley and success is more likely, provided her condition permits, if she is allowed to use a commode and be left alone for a few minutes. The urine is retained for examination.

The patient is then turned on to his left side with the buttocks extending to the edge of the trolley. The nurse supports the patient from his front, requesting him to 'roll into a ball' and 'take a few deep breaths', while the doctor examines the rectum digitally wearing a well-lubricated glove. The presence of blood on the examining finger suggests hemorrhage while tenderness anteriorly on rectal examination may be either due to intraperitoneal hemorrhage or peritonitis arising from a ruptured viscus.

COLLECTION OF URINE

A specimen of urine must be obtained for examination. The patient preferably provides a sample prior to rectal examination but if he is undiagnosed and seriously ill or comatose or otherwise unable to micturate voluntarily he must be catheterized under sterile conditions. A specimen of urine may help towards the diagnosis and in the subsequent management by providing an accurate assessment of renal function.

Catheterization

The decision to catheterize the patient is made by the medical staff and it is their responsibility although nursing personnel may be delegated to pass the catheter.

Technique. The nurse prepares a trolley, placing on the top shelf a catheter pack with sterile towels and bowls, a tube of local analgesic gel with nozzle, antiseptic, syringes, sterile water and lubricating jelly. On the bottom shelf she arranges a sterile receiver, disposable towels, cotton wool swabs, 2 pairs of dissecting forceps, specimen containers and measuring jugs.

Bags are fastened to the trolley side for discarded towels and swabs. The person who is delegated to pass the catheter first thoroughly washes her hands and dries them on a sterile paper towel. The glans penis, or the vulva, is washed with antiseptic solution and sterile towels are arranged around the urethral orifice. The sterile local analgesic gel is inserted into the urethra using the nozzle provided with the tube. In the male, the contents of one tube produce satisfactory analgesia. A penile clamp is applied to prevent loss of the analgesic gel and after a few minutes delay for it to act, sterile gloves are donned and a well-lubricated catheter is gently passed into the bladder.

Type of catheter. A non-indwelling plastic catheter of between 12–16 French gauge is suitable if catheterization is performed to obtain a urinary specimen or demonstrate the integrity of the urinary tract.

An indwelling catheter of the Foley pattern between 14–20 French gauge is the most suitable for continuous drainage (Figure 4.1). This type of catheter is retained in the urinary bladder by a small balloon which is inflated by the injection of sterile water through the side arm. The amount of fluid required for optimal inflation of the balloon is printed on either the packet or side arm of the catheter.

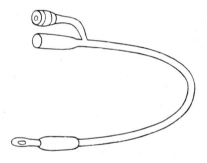

Figure 4.1 Foley catheter

If catheterization is performed for acute retention of urine and there is a long history of urinary difficulties, such as recurring retention and poor urinary flow, decompression of the urinary bladder should be slow because of the risk of severe hemorrhage from the bladder wall.

If the catheter does not pass readily into the bladder or if hemorrhage is encountered, the procedure should be abandoned. In these circumstances if rupture of the urinary tract is suspected, the patient is admitted directly to the operating theatre or ward for attempted catheterization under general anesthesia, followed, if indicated, by operative repair of either the urethra or bladder.

Suprapubic decompression

If the acute retention of urine is unrelieved by the passage of a urethral catheter in the Accident and Emergency department, yet it is obvious that the patient has an intact urethra, the doctor may decompress the bladder by suprapubic puncture. This procedure consists of inserting a long needle, such as a lumbar puncture needle, or a plastic catheter on an introducer into the bladder above the pubic symphysis. A strictly aseptic technique is always necessary when performing suprapubic puncture. Therefore, the nurse assists the doctor and prepares a trolley with lumbar puncture needles and plastic cannulae, local analgesic solution, syringes, needles, antiseptic lotion and sterile gloves. After puncture of the bladder, she attaches a sterile plastic tube to the needle and collects the urine in a plastic bag.

Suprapubic puncture permits emergency decompression of the bladder but is unsuitable for long-term drainage as leakage of urine around the puncture wound in the bladder results in infection of the soft tissues. Any infection which is introduced into the bladder by catheterization may result in pyelonephritis, cystitis or urethritis and additionally in the male, prostatitis, epididymitis or orchitis.

Urine obtained with or without catheterization is examined for blood, protein, sugar and bile, using a Lab-Stick. Urine may be discoloured for a variety of reasons. For example, the ingestion of beets can produce a red-coloured urine imitating hematuria. Therefore, positive evidence of blood in the urine must be obtained before diagnosing hematuria.

FURTHER MANAGEMENT

While the patient remains in the Accident and Emergency department his general condition is regularly observed by the nurse who records his pulse, blood pressure and respiratory rate, in addition to measuring and retaining any vomit or fecal material for examination. The nurse records any change in the conscious level of the patient and alerts the doctor accordingly.

Shock and blood sampling

Patients who have been vomiting for several hours, or who are suffering from hypovolemic shock due to intra-abdominal hemorrhage, require resuscitation. All nursing and medical staff working in the department must be ever alert to the possibility that surgical shock due to loss of circulating blood volume may develop insidiously. A falling blood pressure with an increased pulse rate in a patient who is pale, anxious and sweating presents no difficulty with diagnosis. However, in the early stages of hypovolemic shock, the full clinical picture is not apparent but any increase in the pulse rate or decrease in the blood pressure should be regarded with suspicion and a 20 ml specimen of blood should be obtained immediately by venepuncture. The blood is transferred to three tubes. One tube contains anticoagulant and is sent to the hematology laboratory along with the request for hemoglobin and white cell count estimation. The other two tubes do not contain anticoagulant; one tube is sent to the biochemical laboratory with a request for a biochemical profile, which includes electrolyte and urea estimations. The third tube is sent to the blood transfusion laboratory with a request for grouping and cross-matching. The quantity of blood requested is estimated by assessing the volume of any blood loss and by the clinical condition of the patient. A trolley (cart) should be instantly available containing equipment necessary to start an intravenous infusion.

X-ray examination
Further X-ray investigations may be requested whereupon the nurse should accompany the patient to the X-ray room taking with her a vomit bowl, swabs (pads) and tissues. The radiographs most frequently requested are the erect chest X-ray and the supine film of the abdomen.

The erect chest X-ray will reveal intrathoracic pathology and/or the presence of free gas beneath the diaphragm which signifies the perforation of a viscus with escape of gas and liquid contents into the peritoneal cavity. The abdominal X-ray may reveal distended loops of bowel, radio-opaque calculi in the renal or biliary tract, or a blurred outline of the psoas muscle on either or both sides of the lumbar spine if retroperitoneal bleeding has caused the formation of an hematoma.

Intravenous pyelogram
This radiological diagnostic procedure depends on the ability of the kidney to concentrate and excrete a radio-opaque medium containing iodine. It is performed if the doctor suspects the presence of a renal injury. Before the procedure the patient is asked if he suffers from asthma, hay fever or an allergy to iodine, in which case if the pyelogram *must* be performed, hydrocortisone hemisuccinate 100 mg intravenously is given prior to the administration of the radio-opaque medium.

Sodium iothalamate is the radio-opaque medium in general use. Following its intravenous injection X-rays of the abdomen are obtained at suitable intervals at the discretion of the radiologist. Films will show the renal outline, calyces pelvis, ureter and bladder and it will be possible to establish their integrity.

An intravenous pyelogram therefore gives information regarding renal function and the presence of any renal injury. It also confirms the presence of both kidneys, which is of vital importance in the later management of the patient with a seriously damaged kidney when a nephrectomy may be indicated. If such a procedure is undertaken in the presence of a solitary kidney, death is certain.

PERSONAL PROBLEMS
Occasionally the patient presents with a problem of a personal nature which he does not wish to discuss with the receptionist or the nurse. His emergency document will then have 'wants to see the doctor' written in the 'complaint' column. The nurse must arrange for such patients to be seen alone in the doctor's office or in an examination room.

Two such problems are described below:

(1) Caught in a zip fastener: occasionally a male patient arrives with the loose skin of his penis firmly caught in the teeth of a zipper or slide fastener. Removal of the zipper requires a local analgesic such as 0.5% plain lignocaine (lidocaine), a 10 ml syringe and a fine needle. An embarrassed patient may prefer the female nurse not to be present when the procedure is taking place, but she must be close by in case the doctor needs any further equipment. Occasionally the zipper or damaged skin may have to be cut away and require suturing with fine suture material. A plastic skin spray is used to seal the wound. Circumferential bandaging is avoided if possible otherwise the reactive swelling which usually occurs after damage to the sensitive penile tissues may compromise the circulation.

(2) Foreign bodies in the vagina: the most usual vaginal foreign body is a forgotten tampon or one in which the extracting string has become detached or curled up out of reach. Many women, particularly young girls who have not been menstruating long, are reluctant to explore the vagina with their fingers in order to remove the misplaced object.

For removing a vaginal foreign body a good light is essential. The nurse provides a vaginal speculum, examining gloves, lubricating jelly and a pair of long forceps. The patient preferably lies on her back with her legs drawn up and abducted but if the patient is too embarrassed to adopt this position she is placed curled up on her side as for a digital examination of the rectum or vagina.

The nurse should be present throughout the procedure partly as a chaperone and partly because the patient may need sympathy and reassurance.

(3) Foreign bodies in the rectum: very occasionally a very

embarrassed patient attends with a foreign body in the rectum. Most Accident and Emergency doctors wisely ask the help of the general surgeon, who will probably require a proctoscope and sigmoidoscope.

5

Soft tissue injuries

V. W. BURTON

Soft tissue injuries include injury to the skin, subcutaneous fat, fascia, muscles, ligaments, tendons and occasionally major blood vessels and nerves. The treatment of wounds has been discussed above.

Large hematomata

Injuries to soft tissue, including muscles and tendons, may be due to either direct violence or vigorous muscle contraction. Direct violence, insufficient to produce a fracture of the bone, may result in rupture of blood vessels sufficient in number and size to produce a hematoma, that is, an encysted collection of blood. This hematoma may be large, especially around the buttocks and may contain up to 1 litre of blood which, while rarely developing rapidly enough to cause hypovolaemic shock, may be responsible for anemia especially in the elderly. If extensive soft tissue bruising is noted, the nurse should monitor the patient by regular recording of his pulse and blood pressure.

The skin overlying a hematoma may be devitalized by the injury and by the subsequent increase in tissue tension resulting in the formation of an ulcer. The problem of skin loss complicating blunt violence is commonly encountered in the elderly who frequently develop ulcers especially distal to the knee. These may require split skin grafting to ensure sound healing. A close follow-up of patients with extensive local bruising is essential, and the nurse alerts the doctor if the hematoma is obviously increasing as indicated by stretching of the overlying skin. He may then decide to aspirate the hematoma or evacuate it through a small incision. If the hematoma is very large, the patient is admitted and an adequate search is made under general anesthesia for any possible major vessel rupture which, when discovered, is best ligated.

Examples of hematomata at different sites

SUBUNGAL HEMATOMA

A subungal hematoma is a tense collection of blood beneath the nail caused by haemorrhage from a crush injury of the terminal segment of a finger. Diagnosis is straightforward, there is a history of a blow followed by nail bed tenderness and the appearance of a bruise beneath the nail.

Immediate relief of pain follows evacuation of the hematoma. A sharp hypodermic needle is used to trephine the nail which is first thoroughly cleaned with a spirit solution. The needle is then rotated between finger and thumb with the point centred over the hematoma until the nail is perforated, indicated by the immediate release of blood.

PERIANAL HEMATOMA

Straining at stool may rupture one of the small cutaneous veins close to the anal margin, resulting in a small, tense subcutaneous hematoma which is very painful. Without treatment the hematoma is slowly absorbed over the ensuing week. Immediate relief is obtained by evacuating the hematoma under local analgesia.

The nurse prepares the minor operating theatre and positions the patient on his side with the normal buttock uppermost. If the patient is obese the buttocks can be separated by using 7.5 cm (3 in) adhesive strapping applied to the overhanging buttock, which is lifted and supported by securing the strapping to the operating table.

The area around the hematoma is washed with soap and water, dried, and any long hairs around the swelling are trimmed with scissors. The doctor uses a 1% lignocaine (lidocaine) solution for local analgesia and evacuates the hematoma by incising the swelling using a number 15 scalpel blade. After complete evacuation of the hematoma a small adhesive dressing is applied and the patient told to return for change of dressing the following day.

UPPER LIMB CONTUSION

A contusion of the forearm needs only a local crepe bandage applied evenly to avoid any undue pressure on the underlying skin. The patient is told to keep the arm elevated and rested in a sling for 2 or 3 days and to regularly exercise the fingers and other related joints. To prevent the development of a frozen shoulder, the patient is advised to exercise the joint at least every 2 hours by first abducting the arm fully then raising the hand behind the head to ensure full external rotation of the shoulder, and finally by placing the hand behind the small of the back to ensure full internal rotation.

LOWER LIMB CONTUSION

In lower limb injury a supporting bandage is applied and the patient is advised to keep the affected limb elevated, preferably on a low stool, and to limit walking activities to essential journeys, such as to the toilet.

Supports

The Accident and Emergency nurse should be capable of advising the patient how to manage a stick, crutches or a walking aid, all of which should be available in the department.

Sticks. If the forefoot alone is damaged, a stick held in the contralateral (opposite) hand to the leg injury will provide support. The stick should be of such a length that the elbow is about 10° short of full extension when held in the 'attention' position. The tip of the stick is covered by a non-slip rubber cap. The patient walks bearing part of his weight on the injured extremity but, at the same time, helping to support himself with the contralateral arm through his walking stick.

Crutches. Likewise with crutches, a few words of advice can save the patient hours of experimentation. The patient's body weight should be supported on the hands and not by the axilla, because prolonged pressure in the axilla exerted by the crutch can compress the underlying nerves where they form the brachial plexus. Pressure on the brachial plexus can cause numbness and weakness of the arm which may take several months to recover.

The crutches are adjusted for height. Two possible adjustments of the crutch are available. The first adjustment controls the overall length which should be gauged to leave a 5 cm (2 in) gap between the top of the crutch and the axillary folds. This gap may crudely be estimated by the breadth of three fingers. The second adjustment determines the height of the hand piece from the top of the crutch and this should be arranged so that the patient's body weight is supported by his hands with the elbows extended.

After adjusting the height of the crutches the nurse should demonstrate crutch walking with complete non-weight bearing on her imaginary affected extremity which she flexes at the knee. The nurse first sits down with the crutches placed close by the chair. Then, after standing on the normal leg she positions the crutches beneath the axillae and supports her weight by both arms and the normal leg. She starts a tripedal gait by leading with both crutches which she lifts and moves forward about 0.5 metres (20 in) in front of the normal foot. When the crutches are secure, she relaxes the normal leg and her momentum carries her forward about 0.5 metre (20 in) in front of the crutches where the normal foot is planted firmly on the ground. She advises the patient to keep the knee of the affected limb flexed and the hip extended. However, if the knee is injured and flexion is impossible, the affected limb is held flexed at the hip while crutch walking. A shoe should be worn on the unaffected foot as this gives further clearance for the injured extremity. Before sitting down, the patient should turn around and feel the chair with the backs of his legs and transfer both crutches to one hand. If numbness, weakness or tingling sensations develop in the hands the patient should contact his medical advisors as these symptoms suggest that pressure is developing on the peripheral nerves in the axilla.

Walking frame. The elderly patient frequently manages at home with a walking aid which offers more stability than crutches although it is somewhat more bulky. Care must be taken that progress is not impeded by any gaps in the floor covering or furniture.

Makeshift walking aids. The patient may manage to move around at home using furniture such as a chair, or even a kitchen trolley (cart), as a walking aid, thereby enabling him to maintain his independence.

Climbing stairs. Stairs should be negotiated either by using the stair rail and one crutch or, alternatively and more safely, by the patient sitting on the bottom stair and propelling himself to the top bearing his weight on the buttocks and the unaffected leg.

Muscle injuries
CLASSIFICATION
Muscle injuries may be classified by their site and severity.

Site
    Muscle belly
    Muscle-tendon junction
    Tendon
Severity
    Rupture of a few fibres.
    Complete rupture of a muscle or tendon without displacement.
    Avulsion of a tendon from its bone attachment.

TREATMENT
If the muscle injury is slight with rupture of only a few muscles fibres, local support with either Tubigrip or a crepe bandage helps to prevent the development of a hematoma. However, care must be taken to ensure that the circulation is not embarrassed. Tubigrip is of special use and is available in several diameters suitable for the arm, forefoot, calf and thigh. The Tubigrip should extend well beyond the limits of the injured muscle. For example, if the calf muscles are injured, the Tubigrip is applied from the toes to just below the knee to prevent the development of swelling around the ankle, which inevitably develops if the bandage is confined to the calf alone.

A sling is provided to support the upper limb, whereas a walking aid, either stick or crutch, is indicated if the patient needs assistance in walking. The doctor may refer the patient to a physiotherapist for ultrasound treatment, which may hasten the absorption of a hematoma within the muscle belly and speed the recovery process. The patient is advised to return to the department if discomfort increases in the affected part.

A severe muscle rupture requires a plaster of Paris cast to rest the injured muscle belly for at least 3 weeks. If the calf muscle is damaged a short leg plaster is applied with the foot in plantar flexion. If the quadriceps muscle is damaged, a plaster of Paris cylinder (Figure 5.1), to maintain the knee in extension, is the treatment of choice. The nurse ensures that the patient understands the plaster instructions (p. 74) and if necessary provides a walking aid, or if no help is available at home, she may suggest that the patient remains in the overnight ward. Referral to an orthopedic clinic is advisable as a period of rehabilitation with physiotherapy will be required.

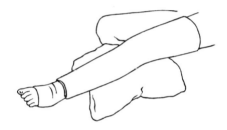

Figure 5.1   Plaster cylinder

MUSCLE-TENDON JUNCTION

The third type of muscle injury, that is complete rupture with displacement, needs open repair with suturing of the muscle to the tendon followed by the application of a protective cast for about 8 weeks. The tendons most commonly injured by violent muscle activity are the Achilles tendon behind the heel and the patellar tendon in front of the knee. A recent rupture of the Achilles tendon may be treated by plaster of Paris cast fixation with the ankle plantar flexed to close the gap between the tendon ends behind the heel. A rupture diagnosed 2–3 days after injury requires surgical repair. A rupture of the patellar tendon should always be treated by surgical repair followed by plaster cast fixation. Both of these tendon injuries require protection in a plaster cast for about 8 weeks.

AVULSION OF THE TENDON ATTACHMENT

A tendon may be avulsed from its attachment to bone by muscle violence. It there is only slight displacement, protection in a suitable splint or plaster cast is indicated. However, a separation which cannot be reduced satisfactorily by manipulation requires open repair by internal fixation.

Common sites for rupture at a tendon insertion

(1) The extensor tendon in the fingers at its attachment to the terminal phalanx.

Avulsion of the tendon results in a mallet finger deformity, (flexion of the terminal interphalangeal joint – Figure 5.2). Treatment with a splint reduces the displacement by holding the interphalangeal joint extended. Provided that such splintage is continued for 6 weeks reattachment of the tendon is achieved with recovery of normal function.

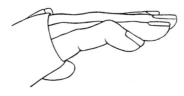

Figure 5.2 Flexion at the terminal interphalangeal joint of the little finger due to rupture of the extensor tendon – 'mallet finger'.

(2) The long head of the biceps muscle at the shoulder.

This occurs especially in the elderly, with haematoma formation and discomfort in the upper arm. The patient should be reassured that normal function of the arm will recover. No active treatment is required except resting the arm in a sling for a few days until the local swelling subsides.

(3) The triceps muscle at its insertion into the tip of the olecranon behind the elbow.

The patient complains of weakness of the elbow with inability to extend the elbow joint. Open repair is necessary as an in-patient.

(4) The patellar tendon attachment to the upper end of the tibia. If there is displacement of the tendon attachment, the patient is unable to extend his knee actively against gravity. These circumstances require admission to hospital and open repair of the tendon.

TENOSYNOVITIS

Tenosynovitis means irritation of the tendon sheath; it is sometimes found in association with a sprained joint when the related tendon has also been damaged. More frequently, however, it occurs following prolonged repetitive movement. For example, involvement of the tendon sheath over the radial aspect of the thumb following excessive activity such as typing, results in local pain, swelling and tenderness on the outer aspect of the wrist.

Treatment
Rest and splintage. Tenosynovitis usually responds to a period of absolute rest either in a plaster cast or splint (Figure 5.3a,b,c) but if the sheaths relevant to the thumb are involved a scaphoid plaster is most suitable (p. 70 and Figure 8.4).

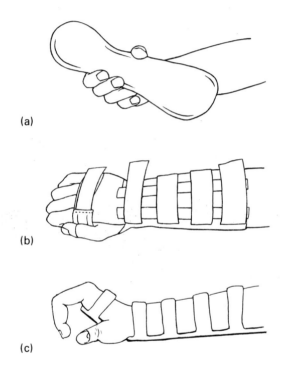

Figure 5.3   Splints:
        (a)   Wrist splint
        (b)   Wrist splint with Velcro fasteners
        (c)   'Cock-up' splint

Steroid infections. If symptoms persist despite 1 or 2 weeks of rest, the tenosynovitis generally responds to a local injection of hydrocortisone or an allied preparation. Various steroid preparations are available:

hydrocortisone acetate (25 mg/ml) or methyl prednisolone acetate (40 mg/ml) are most popular and are usually given in a 2 ml syringe. A local analgesic solution such as lignocaine (lidocaine) 1% should be available because some doctors prefer to inject a mixture of steroid with an analgesic to reduce the local discomfort. The nurse wears a mask, washes her hands and prepares a trolley. Shaving is unnecessary but the skin is washed with soap and water and cleaned with a spirit solution such as chlorhexidine and spirit. A large bore needle such as a size 9 G 50 mm (2 in) needle is used to draw the steroid solution into the syringe, taking full sterile precautions. The needle is changed for a 23 G which the doctor inserts into the affected tendon sheath and injects 1 ml of the steroid preparation. The patient is warned that some discomfort over the affected tendon will occur and last for several hours. The locally instilled steroid reduces the inflammatory response in the tendon sheath and its action continues for about 2 weeks (or longer depending on the preparation). A further injection may be required before complete remission is achieved.

Injuries to nerves

A brief description of nerve injuries is included to stress the importance of testing for an associated nerve injury in every patient who attends the Accident and Emergency unit with a limb injury. Should this vital assessment be omitted and evidence of a nerve injury be found several months after the original accident, it is impossible to assess whether the function of a nerve has improved or deteriorated.

EXAMINATION
A history of the injury is important and it should be recorded whether there has been any contusion, cut or abrasion which may have damaged the peripheral nerve.

Position of the limb
The attitude of the limb may indicate nerve damage; for example, wrist drop which is the flexed attitude of the wrist is seen when the extensor tendons of the wrist are paralyzed because of damage to the radial nerve in the arm. Foot drop describes the plantar flexed attitude of the foot following paralysis of the dorsiflexors of the ankle caused by damage to the lateral popliteal nerve, usually in the region where it is closely related to the head of the fibula on the outer aspect of the knee.

Muscles
If the peripheral nerve is cut immediate loss of muscle power is demonstrated on examination. Later muscles innervated by it become wasted and flabby due to loss of tone.

Sensation
Pain sensation is generally assessed by pin prick, light touch is tested by touching with a portion of cotton, and temperature sense is tested by applying test tubes containing hot and cold water. Most of these sensations are partially or completely lost in the area supplied by the damaged peripheral nerve.

Trophic changes
These changes become apparent several months after nerve injury and are due to loss of vasomotor tone in small blood vessels of the skin causing the skin to become cold and dry with fissure formation. Eventually the nails become brittle and the subcutaneous fat atrophies.

Further information concerning peripheral nerve function is obtained by testing the electrical conduction of nerve using the technique of electromyography.

DIAGNOSIS
As a result of the clinical investigations four syndromes may be identified:

Syndrome of complete interruption
The nerve has been completely divided, there is a complete flaccid paralysis of the muscle groups innervated by the nerve with complete loss of sensation.

Syndrome of incomplete interruption
This syndrome is encountered where the nerve has been damaged possibly by scar tissue or by callus formation from related fractures. There is partial loss of sensation, and although some muscle wasting is evident, some power of voluntary movement is retained.

Syndrome of compression
Compression of a peripheral nerve results in a syndrome of incomplete interruption of impulses in the nerve fibres with the addition of painful paresthesiae. The patient has discomfort and tingling sensations in the cutaneous distribution of the peripheral nerve. If symptoms persist he should be referred to an orthopedic clinic in case surgical decompression of the peripheral nerve is required.

Syndrome of recovery
Some previously absent function of the peripheral nerve may be found on sensory and motor testing. Recovery may be demonstrated by eliciting a positive Tinel's sign which involves tapping over the course of the nerve with the examining finger and producing a tingling sensation

in the cutaneous distribution of the nerve (a positive Tinel's sign). Previously flaccid and paralyzed muscle bellies may be seen to contract before muscle power is capable of moving a related joint.

TREATMENT
If there is an open wound the patient is admitted to hospital and the wound is explored in the main operating theatre. If the nerve has been damaged in a closed injury, complete rest of the paralyzed muscles is advisable. The muscles are splinted in a relaxed position. For example, a wrist drop due to a radial nerve palsy requires a simple cock-up splint to maintain the wrist in extension. If the patient has lost sensation in the fingers a glove is worn for protection against accidental burns.

Neurotmesis
This term indicates complete rupture of the nerve fibres and sheath. There is an anatomical rupture of the nerve and perhaps a wide gap between the divided ends which the natural growth of the fibres will be unable to bridge thereby causing permanent loss of function unless nerve suturing is performed. This injury is encountered in open wounds and occasionally following violent closed injuries to the extremities associated with severe fractures or dislocations.

Axonotmesis
In this injury small fibres within the nerve are ruptured without damaging the continuity of the nerve sheath. The nerve fibres eventually regenerate down the sheath, and function recovers without the need for surgical repair.

Neuropraxia
In this injury the nerve fibres and sheaths remain intact but temporary impairment of nerve function is in evidence following a local contusion, continued pressure or stretching, all of which may be trivial. The interruption of impulse conduction in the nerve is therefore due to a physiological disturbance and not to an anatomical lesion. Initially there is paralysis of muscles and some loss of sensation. The recovery phase starts after a period which varies between hours and weeks.

Examples of neuropraxia. These include compression of the lateral popliteal nerve at the head of the fibula due to a local blow or tight plaster and can cause foot drop. Sitting with the arm over the back of a chair can cause wrist drop due to pressure on the radial nerve where it is closely applied to the humerus. Crutch palsy can also follow compression of the brachial plexus by a crutch in the axilla (p. 38).
These lesions are encountered more frequently in patients with a

history of prolonged unconsciousness following a bout of heavy drinking or an overdose of sedative drugs. A neuropraxia of a peripheral nerve may follow general anesthesia unless care is taken to ensure that no pressure is applied to the tissue overlying any vulnerable peripheral nerve.

The treatment for both an axonotmesis and neuropraxia is the protection of insensitive skin combined with splintage of the extremity in an attempt to prevent over-stretching of the paralyzed muscles. If recovery of nerve function is not obvious after a 3 month period, nerve conduction studies are performed, and if there is then no evidence of nerve fibre regeneration the nerve is exposed by operation.

6

Joint injuries

V. W. BURTON

Joints may be injured by either direct violence, such as in a car crash where the front passenger's flexed knee strikes the dashboard, or by indirect violence when, for example, a footballer injures his knee by twisting it while his foot is held firmly in a studded boot that is stuck in soft ground.

Classification of joint injuries

(1) Ligamentous sprains and ruptures
(2) Internal derangements
(3) Dislocations

LIGAMENTOUS SPRAINS AND RUPTURES

Ligamentous injuries are common. The range of movement of the joint is estimated and compared with the normal side. A joint should not be considered normal unless there is a full range of pain-free movement. If only a few fibres within the ligament are damaged, only local swelling is evident, whereas complete rupture of the ligament causes bleeding into the joint cavity with the formation of a haemarthrosis with a generalized swelling of the joint. Pain and swelling may be localized to the ligament if the injury is a sprain but are more diffuse if there is a hemarthrosis secondary to a ligamentous rupture.

Interphalangeal joints

A sprain of the collateral ligament of the interphalangeal joint of the finger can be adequately protected by strapping the damaged digit to the adjacent normal finger (Figure 6.1). Gauze is placed between the fingers to prevent maceration of the skin and fixation is then achieved by means of a 12.5 mm (0.5 in) zinc oxide strapping applied in 3 hoops, each one centred over the phalanx, the distal hoop being secured to the finger nail. This form of splintage is especially useful as it does permit

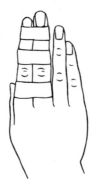

Figure 6.1   Finger strapping

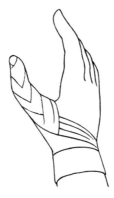

Figure 6.2   Adhesive plaster thumb spica

some movement of the finger joint thereby limiting post-traumatic stiffness.

Sprains of the thumb are treated in a spica fashioned from 2.5 cm (1 in) strips of adhesive strapping (Figure 6.2).

WRIST INJURIES

The diagnosis of a sprained wrist should generally only be made after excluding a fracture. The scaphoid bone, which lies on the radial side of the wrist joint in the proximal row of the carpus, may be fractured by a fall on the outstretched hand causing pain and local tenderness over the radial aspect of the wrist. If a fractured scaphoid is inadequately treated without plaster cast fixation it will not unite. Permanent disability follows and osteoarthritis will almost certainly develop in the wrist at a later date.

Severe ligamentous injuries at the wrist respond to complete rest for 2 or 3 weeks in a short arm plaster cast, whereas sprains of the wrist respond to local splintage. The fingers should be exercised regularly and the hand elevated in a sling for the first 48 hours.

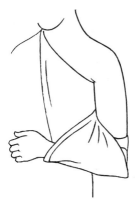

Figure 6.3   Broad arm sling

SHOULDER INJURIES

At the shoulder both the gleno-humeral joint and the acromio-clavicular joint may be injured by either a direct blow to the region or by a heavy fall on the outstretched hand. A broad arm sling (Figure 6.3) is applied to support the weight of the arm, ensuring that the shoulders are level and that the sling is comfortable with plenty of padding, such as gamgee tissue (absorbent wool covered with gauze) around the neck. A so-called frozen shoulder (a condition typified by a painful, stiff shoulder joint) may readily develop after minor shoulder injuries, particularly in the elderly, and therefore early mobilization is recommended (p. 37).

ANKLE INJURIES

A sprain of the lateral ligament of the ankle is very common and is caused by the patient 'going over on the outer border of the foot' when walking on rough ground. Maximal tenderness is present anterior and inferior to the lateral malleolus. An associated ankle fracture should always be excluded by radiological examination.

Treatment is local splintage using adhesive plaster provided that the patient is not allergic to it. The skin is shaved distal to the knee and 'stirrup strapping' is applied to support the damaged ligament as follows – the first bandage is applied at just below the knee down the inner side of the calf and is then carried under the heel, maintaining tension on the strapping until it is firmly secured to the lateral aspect of the calf, thereby applying lateral support to the ankle. Two or three circumferential turns of adhesive plaster anchor the strapping securely to the leg. The plaster may require changing at 10 days and overall should be retained for about 3 weeks. If there is marked swelling of the joint and the patient is unable to stand, alternative treatment consists of a short leg walking plaster cast.

KNEE INJURIES
Knee injuries require expert assessment as soon as possible. As with other joints, ligaments may be sprained or ruptured and intra-articular structures may be torn.

History
The history obtained from the patient is important because a knee injury caused by direct contact suggests there may be ligamentous involvement. For example, a severe blow over the *outer* aspect of the knee followed by pain experienced on the *inner* aspect of the joint suggests damage to its medial collateral ligament. On the other hand, twisting of the knee followed by severe pain localized to one side of the knee joint suggests a torn meniscus. The presence of swelling and its speed of development are important. Immediate swelling after an injury suggests injury to a vascular structure such as bone or ligament and the presence of a haemarthrosis. Damage to an avascular structure, such as a meniscus, also causes joint swelling due to synovial effusion, but this develops slowly over a 24 hour period.

Examination
The clinical examination determines the range of movement and the presence of any haemarthrosis or synovial effusion. The doctor pays particular attention to the stability of the knee and if there is any abnormal movement suggesting complete ligamentous rupture he asks for specialist help and admits the patient for surgical repair.

However, if the stability of the knee is in doubt and/or a hemarthrosis of the knee is suspected but the anteroposterior, lateral and oblique X-rays of the knee are normal, the doctor may decide to aspirate the knee and examine it under general anesthesia.

Joint aspiration
The nurse prepares the Accident and Emergency theatre, and provides packs, towels and a 50 ml syringe with a 14 G aspiration needle.

The first requirement for a safe aspiration is an aseptic technique. The skin is shaved around the knee, which is then washed with soap and water and then cleansed with a spirit based antiseptic solution. Sterile towels are positioned around the knee, leaving the front of the knee joint uncovered. The skin, subcutaneous tissues and synovium are all infiltrated with a 1% lignocaine solution prior to puncture and aspiration of the joint if local analgesia is preferred.

Following withdrawal of the needle, the skin puncture is sealed with a small self-adhesive plaster dressing, followed by the application around the joint of wool and a conforming bandage. If following aspiration and examination a hemarthrosis is confirmed but the ligaments are found to be intact, a plaster of Paris cylinder is applied in order to rest the knee in extension and the patient is then supplied with crutches. If, however, under general anesthesia abnormal movement is demonstrated, indicating a major ligamentous rupture, the patient is admitted to hospital for treatment.

If many fat globules are noted in the aspirated blood, the casualty doctor will suspect an interarticular fracture which was not apparent on the X-rays and requests the opinion of an orthopedic specialist.

Synovial effusion

Minor ligamentous knee injuries and contusions frequently produce a post-traumatic synovial effusion. Treatment with a local supporting bandage consisting of alternate layers of wool and domette (Figure 6.4)

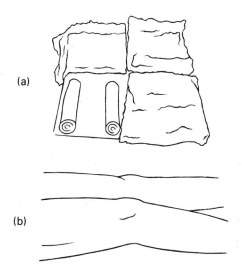

(a)

(b)

Figure 6.4 Supporting knee bandage:
    (a) Layers of wool and domette
    (b) Synovial effusion right knee

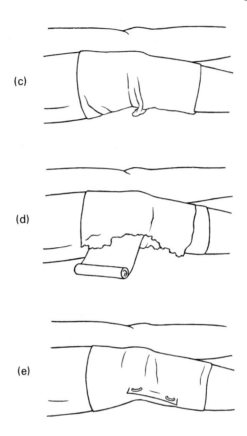

(c)

(d)

(e)

Figure 6.4   (c–e)   Application of alternate layers of wool and domette

relieves pain and hastens recovery. Sticks or crutches are provided and the patient instructed to attend the department for review in 48 hours.

Torn cartilage
A torn meniscus following a rotational knee injury may produce a locked knee, whereupon the patient can neither bend nor straighten the joint, and any attempt to do so evokes severe pain. A synovial effusion is frequently present. The doctor manipulates the knee under general anaesthesia which abolishes the protective muscle spasm so that unlocking is usually and readily achieved. A supporting crepe bandage is applied and crutches or a stick are provided. Arrangements are made for his subsequent follow-up because of the anticipated recurrence of locking of the knee or its 'giving way' with the sensation of insecurity.

ACUTE NECK PAIN

The syndrome of acute cervical pain, possibly with radiation to one or both arms, is not uncommon especially in patients past middle age. Most cases are due to degenerative changes in the cervical spine with irritation of the nerve roots. When conditions such as bone infection, malignancy and dislocations have been excluded and the diagnosis of degenerative disc disease has been substantiated, a cervical collar is applied to support the patient's head and neck. A convenient collar is made from covering a shaped piece of cardboard with wool and stockinette (Figure 6.5). There should be one finger's breadth of clearance between the chin and top of the collar. The patient is referred back to his practitioner, or Physical Medicine department if he requires physiotherapy treatment.

DISLOCATIONS

Dislocations are inevitably associated with extensive ligamentous injury. Treatment consists of reduction of the dislocation as soon as is practicable and immobilization to promote healing of the soft tissues.

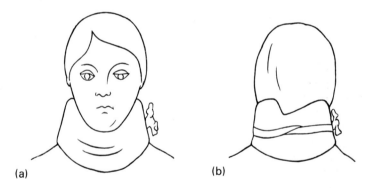

(a)   (b)

Figure 6.5 (a & b) Cervical collar made of cardboard and covered with stockinette

However, some dislocations, especially those encountered at the ankle, are accompanied by fractures involving the articular surface. These injuries are treated in the major operating theatre because they require an accurate open reduction and internal fixation of the fracture.

Common dislocations encountered in the Accident and Emergency department are at the interphalangeal joints of the fingers, at the elbow (Figure 6.6.), shoulder or temporomandibular joint and occasionally at the hip joint.

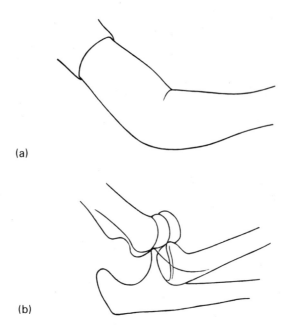

(a)

(b)

Figure 6.6   Posterior dislocation of elbow:
        (a)   Appearance of the arm
        (b)   The relationship of the humerus to the radius and ulna

As with all major limb injuries the neurological status must be evaluated. Frequently the brachial plexus is injured by the head of the humerus in a shoulder dislocation, the ulnar nerve in an elbow dislocation and the sciatic nerve in a posterior dislocation of the hip. The vascular status of the limb must also be assessed by observing the colour of either the hand or foot and noting the presence of the peripheral pulses distal to the discolouration.

The nurse assists the doctor to undress the patient and carry out his examination. Care and patience are essential. She supports his injured extremity at all times and applies a temporary sling if the upper limb is involved, and a temporary 'Jet' splint (Figure 6.7) when the ankle joint is injured if the deformity suggests the presence of a dislocation. A 'Jet splint' is an inflatable splint with a zip fastener which makes it simple to apply. After its application the splint is inflated by a small hand pump until its outer skin is convex. The criticism usually directed towards this form of splint is that it may compress the peripheral veins and possibly encourage thrombosis. An alternative temporary splint is a 'Vac Pac'

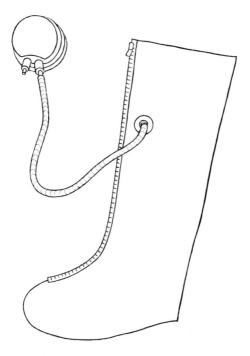

Figure 6.7 Jet splint

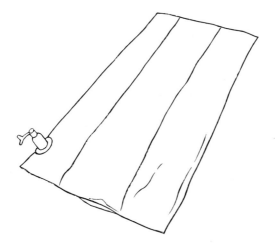

Figure 6.8 'Vac Pac'

(Figure 6.8) which consists of a washable material shaped like a pillow containing a large number of polystyrene granules. The splint is moulded gently around the injured limb. Then a negative pressure is applied to the splint by means of a portable suction machine which removes all air between the granules, transforming them into a rigid compact mass that immobilizes the injured extremity.

Inflatable splints and Vac Pacs are satisfactory for the temporary splintage of injuries in the lower extremity, distal to the thigh; they do not impair the quality of a radiograph. The doctor prescribes an analgesic which is administered by the nurse, generally by intramuscular injection (p. 19).

Reduction of any dislocation should be performed as soon as possible. Many finger dislocations may be reduced without the use of an anesthetic. A larger joint such as the elbow (Figure 6.9) requires the relaxation achieved by general anesthesia unless there is a contraindication (p. 105) to the administration of a general anesthetic. The

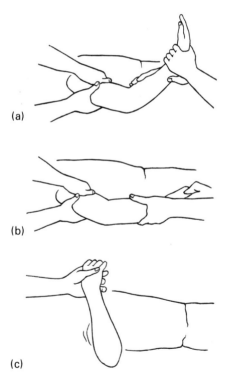

Figure 6.9   Elbow dislocation reduced by manipulation

nurse prepares a collar and cuff (Figure 6.10) for elbow injuries and a broad arm sling (Figure 6.3) for shoulder injuries.

Hip dislocations are occasionally reduced in the department. Considerable force may be required to reduce a posterior dislocation which can only be exerted by the surgeon if the patient is anesthetized on a mattress on the floor. Following reduction of a hip dislocation, the patient is admitted to hospital and the reduction is maintained by traction.

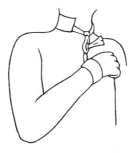

Figure 6.10 Collar and cuff

Traction
Traction may be applied to the skin by a self-adhesive plaster, when it is described as skin traction, or it may be applied by a metal nail transfixing the tibia, when it is known as skeletal traction.

A nurse may be asked to apply the skin traction. The limb is shaved from the groin to the ankle and the skin painted with tinc.benz.co., to enhance the adhesive properties of the plaster. A small 5 cm (2 in) cotton bandage is wrapped around the limb at the level of the head of the fibula to protect the lateral popliteal nerve which, being closely adherent to bone in this region, can be damaged by prolonged traction on the overlying skin. Following application of the adhesive plaster to both sides of the limb, a supporting crepe bandage is wrapped around the limb from the ankle to the groin. The patient is then admitted to the ward and traction applied to the limb by slinging the traction cords over a pulley and attaching a weight to their ends.

7

Fractures

V. W. BURTON

A bone may be injured by direct or indirect violence. A force acting directly on the bone, such as a car bumper striking the tibia, may cause local bleeding and the development of a subperiosteal hematoma.

A force acting on the extremity sufficiently powerful to break the bone causes a fracture in the area of optimum stress. Some patients are more liable to fracture than others; the elderly are especially prone because of the osteoporosis which inevitably develops with increasing age.

Transverse, spiral and oblique are terms used to describe different kinds of fractures. The nature of the violence which has caused the injury may be identified by the type of fracture. If the direction of the deforming force is identified reduction of the fracture should be attempted by applying force in the opposite direction.

Direct violence generally produces a transverse fracture, while indirect violence produces a spiral fracture. For example a spiral fracture occurs when rotational forces act on the tibia of a footballer who twists his knee suddenly with his foot firmly fixed to the ground by a studded boot.

Classification of fractures

(1) *Closed (simple)*
   The fracture hematoma does not communicate with the exterior.
(2) *Open (compound)*
   The fracture hematoma communicates with the exterior, either through the skin or mucous membrane. The diagnosis of an open fracture is important because of the risk of bone infection.
(3) *Comminuted*
   This term indicates shattering of the bone and is generally associated with severe trauma.

(4) *Greenstick*

This type of fracture occurs in young children when one cortex of the bone is fractured leaving the opposite cortex intact, causing bowing of the bone.

(5) *Complicated*

There is damage to associated blood vessels, nerves and organs. For example, the supracondylar fracture of the humerus in children can damage the brachial artery in front of the elbow. A fracture of the left 11th rib can damage the spleen, resulting in a hemoperitoneum.

(6) *Pathological*

This fracture occurs through abnormal bone. There may be a bone cyst, primary or secondary tumour, or localized infection of the bone which renders it more liable to fracture.

(7) *Stress*

In the absence of a single traumatic incident, bone may fracture as the result of continued stress, rather akin to metal fatigue. Such a fracture may be found in a metatarsal or in the upper tibial shaft.

Fracture diagnosis

Fractures are diagnosed by obtaining a good clinical history and performing an adequate examination. The nurse can frequently obtain vital information which leads to the diagnosis of a fracture by obtaining a history from the patient himself or from his relatives, onlookers or the police. If there is a history of a violent injury, such as a motor cycle crashing at speed, the nurse should suspect multiple fractures, particularly those of the spine and pelvis which may not be as clinically obvious as fractures of the femora and tibiae. A less dramatic history from an elderly patient who falls on the outstretched hand, followed by pain and deformity at the wrist (Figure 7.1) with loss of function, suggests that there is a fracture in the region of the wrist joint.

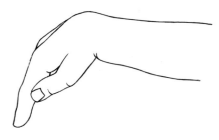

Figure 7.1　Wrist deformity associated with a Colles' fracture

FRACTURE SYMPTOMS

The nurse may suspect a possible serious skeletal injury from the patient's initial complaint. For example, the elderly lady who has fallen, injuring her hip, may complain of discomfort at the fracture site but her most pressing problem is her inability to walk. Similarly, the patient with a fracture around the wrist joint complains that the hand is useless and weak.

The nurse is, therefore, frequently able to make a diagnosis on her first contact with the patient.

FRACTURE SIGNS

The physical signs of a fracture include local bruising and swelling due to rupture of small blood vessels. Local tenderness may be elicited especially where a bone such as the tibia or ulna is subcutaneous. If the fracture is displaced, deformity is evident. Crepitus, a creaking sensation, may be apparent at the site of fracture when the affected limb is moved. Crepitus is due to the fragmented bone surfaces rubbing together and it is a certain diagnostic sign of fracture. However, there should be no attempt made to elicit this sign as movement at the fracture site increases blood loss, results in increased local pain and possibly increases the degree of shock.

After 2 or 3 days, local blisters may develop due to ischaemia of the skin overlying the fracture. Their appearance should alert the medical and nursing personnel to the possible presence of an underlying and possibly missed fracture.

FRACTURE COMPLICATIONS

Vessels and nerves may be injured. For example, a supracondylar fracture of the humerus (Figure 7.2) above the elbow joint, commonly encountered in children, may damage either the brachial artery or the median nerve. The circulation is therefore monitored closely while the

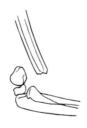

Figure 7.2   Supracondylar fracture of the humerus. Posterior displacement of the distal fragment of the humerus. Manipulative reduction required

patient is in the Accident and Emergency department. The colour and capillary return to the finger tips are noted and the radial pulse palpated. If there is brachial artery compression, local pain is experienced, the fingers may be white or cyanosed and the radial pulse absent. If treatment by urgent reduction of the fracture and possible exploration of the artery restoring the blood flow to normal is delayed, a Volkmann's ischemic contracture due to necrosis of the flexor muscle mass in the forearm develops with contracture of all the fingers. Therefore, the nurse must be ever alert to the possibility of ischemia developing in an extremity following a fracture. If a plaster cast has been applied, it should be bivalved immediately to ensure that there is no pressure from the cast on the underlying skin over the front of the elbow. Apart from the appearance of the fingers and the complaint of pain, the earliest sign that an ischemic contracture is developing is limitation of passive extension of the fingers. The nurse should therefore report any loss of finger joint extension to the doctor especially where the victim has sustained a supracondylar fracture or fracture of both bones in the forearm.

Neurogenic shock

Apart from the local signs and symptoms of fracture, other generalized phenomena may be noted. Neurogenic 'shock' (p. 140) due to pain is frequently encountered even in minor fractures such as those involving the finger phalanges. The patient perspires, is pale and may feel faint and nauseated. Neurogenic shock develops suddenly and is due to pooling of the blood in small vessels which have become dilated due to reflex activity. There is therefore a deficient return of blood to the heart resulting in a reduced cardiac output with consequent tachycardia and hypotension.

The patient suffering from neurogenic shock without blood or fluid loss should be nursed lying down, any fractures adequately splinted and pain relieved by intramuscular morphine, unless there is a significant head injury. Body heat is conserved by the application of blankets but extraneous heat from hot water bottles is better avoided. If the patient still feels faint despite these measures, the foot of the trolley (gurney) should be elevated.

Hypovolemic shock

Hypovolemic shock (p. 139) due to loss of circulating blood volume frequently complicates major fractures. For example, 1.7 litres (3 pints) of blood may be lost into the soft tissues of the thigh following a fracture of the femur, while double that quantity may be lost to the circulation in an extensive fracture of the pelvis. The patient is anxious and pale, respirations are shallow and rapid, the pulse rate is increased and the blood pressure is low. The measures already described in the treatment of neurogenic shock should be instituted immediately by starting an intravenous infusion which should include the transfusion of compatible blood as soon as is practicable.

INVESTIGATION
The clinical diagnosis of fracture or dislocation must be confirmed by X-ray examination. Films of the affected bone or joint should be obtained in two planes, that is an anteroposterior view as well as a lateral view, because fractures may not be visible on a single projection. The joints above and below the suspected fracture should be visible on the X-ray as associated dislocations and subluxations of related joints are often encountered, especially in the forearm and in the leg distal to the knee. For example, the displaced or angulated fracture of the lower third of the radius with an intact ulna may be associated with a dislocation of the inferior radio-ulnar joint.

The patient should be adequately splinted prior to X-ray examination, upper limb injuries should be supported in a sling or held more rigidly in a Vac-Pac. Fractures around the ankle or tibia are splinted.

Fractures of the femur cannot be adequately controlled by a simple splint because of the bulky thigh muscles and the presence of marked limb shortening. The shortening may be overcome by traction to the leg which aligns the fracture. It is our policy to apply a Thomas' splint immediately the clinical diagnosis of a fractured femur is made. The Thomas' splint (Figure 7.3) consists of a padded ring, through which the leg is threaded, and two lateral bars which lie on opposite sides of the leg. Slings are used to support the leg and traction is exerted through adhesive straps applied to the skin on both sides of the leg.

Application of Thomas' splint
The trolley (cart) is prepared having on its top shelf skin extension strapping, shaving equipment, tinc.benz.co., elastic bandages, safety pins and a tension bar.

On the bottom shelf are domette slings, cottonwool and a support for the Thomas splint.

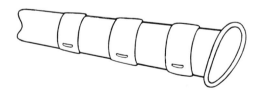

Figure 7.3   Thomas splint with three canvas slings secured with safety pins

The doctor supports the limb by applying traction to the foot and maintaining the leg in neutral rotation.

The nurse measures the circumference of the thigh at the level of the greater trochanter and adds another 4 cm (1.5 in) to allow for any further swelling of the thigh. The nurse then measures from the greater trochanter to the plantar aspect of the foot and adds a further 20 cm (8 in) to allow plenty of space for the skin extension cords to be fixed to the bottom of the splint.

If the patient is conscious the procedure is explained to him. The limb is shaved from groin to ankle. A cotton bandage 7.5 cm (3 in) wide is applied to the knee at the level of the head of the fibula to protect the lateral popliteal nerve from possible traction injury. The skin extension strapping is then applied to both the medial and lateral aspects of the limb. The doctor or nurse supports the limb and applies gentle longitudinal traction by holding the ankle with the fingers and supporting the Achilles tendon, while the other hand simultaneously supports the knee. The second operator then applies the splint, threading the ring over the foot and passing it upwards until the medial portion of the padded ring abuts against the ischial tuberosity of the patient's pelvis. The traction cords are fixed to the plaster adhesive and then carried over and under the lateral bars of the splint before being firmly tied to the end of the splint.

The first operator continues her longitudinal traction of the limb supporting the knee while slings are placed in position behind the thigh and calf. A small pad of wool is placed behind the knee to ensure 5° of flexion at this joint.

After application of the Thomas splint its ring should rest gently against the ischial tuberosity. The limb should lie in a neutral rotation with the anterior superior iliac spine, patella and great toe in alignment. The colour, sensation and active movements of the toes should all be noted. If there is any suggestion of circulatory embarrassment the doctor must be informed immediately.

The patient may now be moved for X-ray examination or for admission into hospital. The skin traction applied to the limb through the adhesive bandage and padded wool gives sufficient support for the fracture for several days. Definitive treatment, possibly converting the traction to skeletal traction using a metal nail through the tibia, or possible operative internal fixation of the fracture, can be undertaken at a later date once the patient's general condition is more stable.

Compound fractures are not managed in the Accident and Emergency department because of the ever present risk of infection. The wound is covered by sterile dressings and the patient admitted to hospital for wound excision.

Fractures which are managed in the department on an out-patient basis include most of the uncomplicated fractures in the upper limb and fractures with minimal displacement in the lower limb, excluding femoral fractures.

Reduction of fractures

After first aid treatment with splintage and X-ray examination the doctor decides whether or not the position of the fracture fragments is acceptable. If the fracture is in an *acceptable* position, a plaster cast is applied. Two operators are required, one to support the injured limb while the other applies the cast. Unless there is a contraindication the joint should be splinted in the position of function. For example, the wrist is splinted with 10° of extension and the ankle with the foot at right angles to the leg.

If the fracture involves the middle of the shaft of a bone, the joint above and below the fracture should be immobilized in a cast. For example, fractures of the midshaft of the forearm bones of children are treated in a long arm cast, likewise fractures of the midshaft of the tibia are treated in a long leg cast.

If the fracture is close to the joint, as in a Colles' fracture of the wrist or a fracture of the lateral malleolus of the ankle, adequate fixation is achieved with either a forearm plaster or a short leg cast.

If the position of the fragments is *unacceptable*, reduction of the fracture is undertaken. Many fractures are reduced by closed manipulation in the Accident and Emergency department under general anesthesia, followed by immobilization of the fracture fragments in a plaster cast.

COLLES' FRACTURE (see also p. 69)
The fracture most frequently reduced in the Accident and Emergency department is the Colles' fracture, in which the lower end of the radius is displaced dorsally and radially. Minor degrees of displacement may be accepted but if angulation is greater than 10°, reduction is indicated especially in young patients. General anesthesia is preferable to local analgesia. The nurse acts as an assistant steadying the arm while the doctor reduces the fracture by disimpacting the fragments by traction followed by correction of the angulation by flexing the wrist and holding it in slight ulnar deviation.

The doctor then holds the wrist in the reduced position by steadying the elbow and holding the little and ring fingers with the wrist slightly flexed while the nurse applies the plaster slab to the padded forearm. The doctor moulds the setting plaster to the contour of the limb applying pressure with the palms of his hands. A wet cotton bandage holds the cast to the forearm.

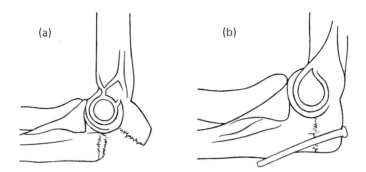

Figure 7.4 (a) Displaced fracture of the olecranon
(b) Accurate reduction and internal fixation with a screw

A sling is applied and once the patient is fully conscious, he is advised to move the fingers regularly and exercise his shoulder every 1 or 2 hours. If the circulation and sensation in the fingers are normal he can return home with an appointment for a plaster check in a fracture clinic on the following day. He will require follow-up for several weeks with one or two plaster changes and a total period of cast fixation until union of the fracture is established in approximately 6 weeks.

Certain fractures cannot be treated adequately by closed manipulation. Displacement may persist due to muscle pull despite manipulation. For example, a fracture through the olecranon at the elbow (Figure 7.4a) disrupts the joint surfaces and displacement persists due to the pull of the triceps musculature. Open reduction and internal fixation (Figure 7.4b) is the treatment of choice following referral for specialist opinion.

8

Plaster technique

V. W. BURTON

Plaster room

The plaster room is an integral part of any Accident and Emergency department. In small district hospitals the plaster facilities are shared by the orthopedic and the accident departments. This concentration of work generally merits the employment of a plaster technician who, with the assistance of the medical and nursing staff, is responsible for the application, removal and repair of casts during normal working hours. At other times the Emergency nurse is expected to apply the plaster casts and splints that are used in the treatment of fractures.

A knowledge of plaster techniques is therefore important for all nursing personnel working in the Accident and Emergency department. There is no substitute for experience. Frequent visits to the plaster room when the plaster technician is present, should be part of a nurse's introduction so that she becomes familiar with the equipment and with the storage areas containing stockinette, plaster wool and plaster of Paris bandages.

The standard cast used in the United Kingdom is based on an open weave plaster of Paris impregnated bandage. Plaster of Paris is anhydrous calcium sulphate which turns into a crystalline mass on the application of water. Therefore, plaster must always be stored in dry surroundings, most of the proprietary bandages being sealed in paper packets. After dipping in water, the bandage adopts a paste-like consistency which makes it ideal for moulding as a splint on to an extremity.

EQUIPMENT REQUIRED IN THE PLASTER ROOM

The plaster room should contain a sink and the floor should be washable. A smooth table top is required for the preparation of plaster slabs. A couch and small stool are necessary for the patient and a small table is useful to support an upper limb while the plaster cast is applied. Cotton sheets and plastic drapes are used to protect the patient's clothes and an apron and boots to protect those of the operator.

Two buckets (pails) supported on a stand at waist height are three-quarters filled with water before plastering starts. One bucket is reserved for dipping bandages whereas the other is used for washing the operator's hands. Other essential items are stockinette, plaster wool, plaster bandages in various widths, plaster slabs, cotton bandages, slings and walking heels. Instruments required in the plaster room include a plaster knife, plaster shears, spreaders, plaster benders and an electrically powered saw.

The forthcoming procedures are explained to the patient and his clothing should be protected.

Plaster cast application
For application of an upper limb cast the patient should be seated comfortably with the affected limb supported on a small table. In lower limb injuries, requiring either a long or a short leg plaster, the patient lies supine on the couch with the affected limb supported by an assistant. In the case of a short leg plaster, the extremity is flexed at the knee over the end of the couch with the foot still being supported either by the operator or by an assistant.

With dry hands, the operator removes the plaster bandages from the airtight packet and arranges them on a smooth surface close to the plaster buckets. Generally cold water is used; the warmer the water the shorter is the setting time. However, if the water temperature is too high the plaster becomes cohesive and will 'layer' with each additional plaster application instead of adhering to the one previously applied, resulting in the production of a weak cast. The water in the plaster dipping bucket should be between 20° and 25°C.

Most casts applied to the limb in the Accident and Emergency department should be padded to allow for subsequent swelling in the soft tissues. Therefore, after placing the limb in the best position for prolonged fixation of the individual injury, a layer of stockinette is first applied, ensuring that there are no areas of constriction, paying particular attention to the base of the thumb and the front of the elbow. A plaster wool bandage is then evenly applied, to avoid any wrinkles and 'build-up' of material over the flexor aspects of the joints such as the elbow, which might constrict the limb and possibly compromise the circulation. Throughout the application of this padding for a long arm cast and, to a lesser extent a long leg cast, the desired degree of flexion anticipated in the final position of the limb must be established and carefully maintained; if padding is applied with the limb extended, subsequent flexion of the elbow to 90°, or the knee to 30°, results in pressure being exerted either on the cubital fossa in front of the elbow, or on the popliteal fossa behind the knee. The effect is a possible compression of either the brachial or popliteal arteries and a certain compression of the veins, which produces further swelling of the limb distal to the joint.

The padding should not be bulky and the overlap with every turn of the bandage is kept to half the bandage width, so that only two layers of plaster wool are applied on top of the stockinette. Excessive use of padding results in a loose cast.

The plaster of Paris bandages are now applied to the limb. It is difficult to find the end of a wet plaster so prior to dipping in the water about 5 cm (2 in) of the bandage is unravelled. The bandage is held at an angle of about 40° (and never vertically) in the bucket, to prevent loss of plaster of Paris from the woven bandage. Immersion continues until all bubbling has ceased. On removal from the bucket, the plaster bandage is squeezed gently to remove excess water. The bandage is then applied in a circumferential manner, each layer being smoothed during its application by the palms of both hands. The plaster is 'unrolled' on to the limb rather than pulled tight. The operator should keep his hands wet and free from hard lumps of plaster by regularly dipping the hands in the second bucket. The required thickness of the plaster cast varies according to its site of application. In the forearm, four layers are sufficient, while a walking short leg plaster requires double this thickness. Care is taken to ensure an adequate thickness of plaster at both ends of the cast. Once the required thickness has been achieved, the ends of the plaster cast are trimmed. With upper limb injuries the patient should be able to flex his fingers fully and in the lower extremity the tips of all the toes should be visible. If the forearm has been immobilized in a plaster cast, the operator must ensure that full flexion can be achieved at the elbow without compression of the skin by the edge of the plaster.

The wet cast must be handled carefully and supported by a pillow wrapped in plastic until it has set. Heat is given off by the drying cast and the patient is warned that the plaster will feel warm. Later the water retained in the plaster cast evaporates and cools the limb. Although the cast sets after 5 minutes if cold water is used, the tensile strength is not maximal until all the water has evaporated, which can take up to 48 hours. Therefore, if a walking plaster is applied, the patient is warned not to put his weight on the cast until this period has passed.

PLASTER CASTS COMMONLY USED
The short arm plaster
This type of cast is applied to the forearm with the wrist in 10° of extension and reaches to the knuckles of the hand (Figure 8.1). It is indicated in severe sprains of the wrist, undisplaced fractures around

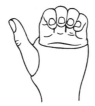

Figure 8.1   Distal end of short arm plaster

the wrist, fractures of the metacarpals and minor undisplaced fractures of the carpal bones. Three 10 cm (4 in) plaster of Paris bandages are required for the average size patient.

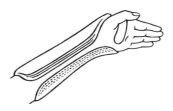

Figure 8.2   Colles' plaster

The Colles' plaster (see also p. 64)
The Colles' plaster is applied to the forearm (Figure 8.2) with the wrist flexed to 10° and deviated to the ulnar side. As the name implies the main indication for its use is the treatment of the Colles' fracture which involves the radius and possibly the ulna, close to the wrist joint. There is often dorsal displacement of the fragments which require manipulative reduction before the application of plaster. Six thicknesses of 20 cm (8 in) plaster bandage in the form of a slab are applied to the dorsal and radial aspects of the forearm (Figure 8.3). A wet 7.5 cm (3 in) cotton bandage maintains the slab in position.

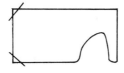

Figure 8.3   Slab for Colles' plaster cut to shape from a 20 cm (8 in) roll

Scaphoid plaster

The principal indication for this plaster cast is a fracture of the scaphoid bone. The wrist and proximal two joints of the thumb are immobilized in the cast until there are clinical and radiological signs of union. Union is frequently rather slow and cast fixation for periods up to 10 weeks are commonplace before the local tenderness over the outer aspect of the wrist resolves, and X-rays confirm union by the disappearance of the gap between the fractured surfaces.

The cast is a modification of the short arm plaster. The wrist is held in 10° of extension and the plaster is continued over the thumb to the level of the inter-phalangeal joint. The thumb is immobilized in such a position of flexion and opposition that the index fingertip and end of the thumb may co-apt (Figure 8.4).

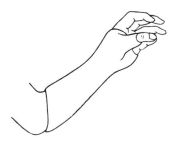

Figure 8.4 Scaphoid plaster

The forearm portion of the cast is applied first, followed by the thumb hand extension which is conveniently made from a series of four or five small plaster slabs 10 cm (4 in) long, 2.5 cm (1 in) wide and four layers thick. These slabs are fashioned from a 10 cm (4 in) plaster bandage.

U slab

This cast is used in the management of fractures of the shaft of the humerus.

The patient is seated, and after adequate analgesia, the arm is supported by an assistant. The fracture is reduced by gentle traction on the elbow which is flexed at 90°.

An oblong portion of orthopedic felt 15 cm (6 in) by 7.5 cm (3 in) is applied to the shoulder; the elbow and arm are padded with orthopedic wool (Figure 8.5).

A 20 cm (8 in) slab ten layers thick is applied to the orthopedic felt, round the elbow to the axilla and secured with a wet cotton bandage. A collar and cuff support the wrist.

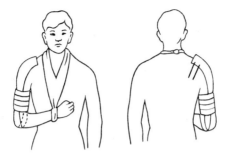

Figure 8.5 U slab

Long arm plaster

The long arm cast is applied to the arm with the elbow bent at a right angle and extends to the knuckles of the hand (Figure 8.6). It is indicated for fractures of the radius and ulna and for fractures at the lower end of the humerus.

Two 15 cm (6 in) and two 10 cm (4 in) plaster bandages are required with the addition of a reinforcing slab consisting of five thicknesses of either a 15 cm (6 in) or a 20 cm (8 in) bandage for reinforcement at the elbow.

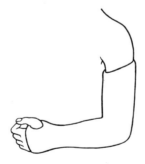

Figure 8.6 Long arm cast

The short leg plaster

The short leg cast is applied to the leg distal to the knee and extends to the toes with the ankle at a right angle.

It is used in the treatment of ankle fractures either undisplaced or for displaced fractures which have been reduced.

Four 20 cm (8 in) and two 10 cm (4 in) plaster bandages are required. The 10 cm (4 in) plaster bandage is applied to the foot and heel. A

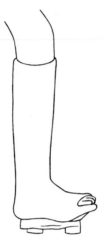

Figure 8.7   Short leg walking plaster

reinforcing slab comprising six thicknesses of a 20 cm (8 in) plaster is also applied, starting under the foot and extending upwards to the midcalf. If the fracture is stable the doctor may incorporate a walking heel which he attaches to the sole of the plaster using a small plaster slab (Figure 8.7). He ensures that the walking heel is positioned below and at a right angle to the vertical axis of the leg, well posteriorly on the sole of the cast. Finally a 10 cm (4 in) plaster bandage secures the walking heel to the cast.

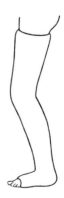

Figure 8.8   Long leg plaster

The long leg plaster

The long leg cast is applied to the leg and extends from the groin to the toes with the ankle at a right angle and the knee slightly flexed at 10° (Figure 8.8). It is indicated for fractures of the tibia and the fibula and for sprains of the ligaments of the knee. The application of this type of cast requires the help of an assistant.

Ten 20 cm (8 in) bandages are wrapped around the leg and the two 10 cm (4 in) bandages around the foot and heel. A reinforcing slab of six thicknesses of 20 cm (8 in) plaster is applied, beginning at the 'ball' of the foot and extending to the mid-calf. A further reinforcing plaster slab may be required at the knee. During application the position of both the knee and the ankle has to be maintained, and the assistant is asked to steady the leg with the knee in the desired position of flexion.

When supporting a limb encased in wet plaster the hands should be wet but only the palms should be used otherwise pressure from a finger tip can cause a pressure sore. The other duty of the assistant is to help mould the plaster to the contour of the leg.

Plaster cylinder

The plaster cylinder is applied to the leg from the groin to above the malleoli at the ankle with the knee extended. It is indicated for undisplaced fractures of the patella, for sprains of the ligaments around the knee and for traumatic synovitis of the knee.

Adhesive plaster straps are first applied to the medial and lateral aspects of the leg followed by a ring of orthopedic felt immediately

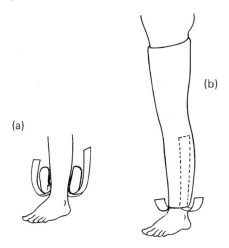

(a)

(b)

Figure 8.9 Plaster cylinder. Adhesive strapping and adhesive felt protecting the skin above the ankle and supporting the cast

above the malleoli (Figure 8.9a). After padding the limb, the cast is applied using six 10 cm (8 in) plaster bandages. The ends of the adhesive straps are turned upwards and together with the orthopedic felt are incorporated in the plaster, so preventing the plaster cylinder from becoming loose and slipping on to the dorsum of the foot (Figure 8.9b).

AFTER-CARE OF THE PLASTER

Before any patient leaves the department wearing a plaster cast he receives a follow-up appointment and printed instructions regarding the care of his cast and warning him of the possible complications which could develop.

Patients attending the Accident and Emergency department in Lancaster receive the following instructions:

(1) Do not leave the hospital without the permission of either the casualty doctor or the charge nurse.
(2) On returning home, drying of the plaster should be continued. You are advised to help this process by sitting by the fire or radiator and then by leaving the plaster uncovered whilst in bed.
(3) Do not bear weight on a leg plaster until permission has been given. Weight bearing is generally permissible after 48 hours.
(4) If the fingers or toes of the injured limb become discoloured (blue or white), cold, swollen or numb, or if the feeling of 'pins and needles' develops, return at once to hospital.
(5) Keep your plaster dry.
(6) Return to the department if the plaster becomes soft or broken.
(7) If in any doubt at any time, return either to your own doctor or to hospital.

The nurse should ensure that the patient understands the instructions before he leaves the hospital.

Finally the nurse arranges a suitable walking aid for the patient and informs him how to protect his plaster from the rain by shielding it in a plastic bag, and how to prevent it soiling the bed clothes by covering it with an old stocking (hose).

CAST REMOVAL

Most casts are removed by bivalving, that is by splitting the plaster cast down both sides with plaster shears or an electric oscillating saw. Plaster shears are preferable when removing casts from children because the electric saw is noisy and perhaps frightening. If there is no padding between the cast and the skin, shears should be used because an oscillating saw may damage the skin.

Use of plaster shears

The plaster shears should be sharp and free of plaster debris. The stockinette extending over the edge of the plaster is cut by scissors and then the shears are inserted, keeping the stockinette between the patient's skin and the instrument. The blade of the shears is always kept parallel to the skin and is advanced after each successive cut of the cast, taking care not to pinch the skin. Special care is needed when dividing the plaster close to any bony protruberance, such as the ankle, where the skin may easily be damaged. In this region it is safer to cut the plaster cast by going behind and below the malleoli.

From time to time the shears become clogged with plaster debris or wool and require cleaning. If difficulty is experienced in reinserting the shears the plaster benders or spreaders are used to increase the gap. Once the plaster is bivalved, the stockinette is cut by scissors and the limb removed from the posterior shell.

Plaster saw

The electric plaster saw cuts plaster by means of an oscillating action but despite this function, laceration of the skin is possible if the instrument is abused. Another disadvantage of the standard electric cutter is that it generates a great deal of dust but a design is now available which incorporates a portable vacuum cleaner.

The operator should demonstrate the saw to the patient, explaining to him that it is noisy and he will experience some vibration while it is in use. Initially the edge of the cast should be divided by scissors because the saw tears rather than cuts the stockinette. The plaster is cut by applying pressure with the edge of the circular saw in repeated small steps at right angles to the limb rather than in a continuous longitudinal cut which is more likely to lacerate the skin. The friction between the blade and plaster produces heat and if the patient experiences discomfort, the saw should immediately be switched off.

Plaster window

If the patient experiences discomfort beneath the plaster, or if the cast becomes offensive with evidence of a discharge, the doctor may ask the nurse to cut a window in the cast. The electric saw is the most satisfactory implement for doing this but before she cuts the window she should mark the projected area clearly with a pencil. The portion of plaster removed is retained as it may be reincorporated in the plaster after the underlying skin has received attention.

Alternative cast materials
There are now available many alternatives to plaster of Paris. The advantages of acrylic acid polymers and the new thermoplastic materials are numerous. For example, their drying time is generally shorter and the thermoplastic materials can be reheated and modelled again; they are stronger and most have washable properties. One major disadvantage is their cost but this can be partly offset by the increased longevity of the cast. They are usually reserved for situations where prolonged treatment is anticipated or for those patients who are 'plaster-bashers'.

Rehabilitation
The patient's rehabilitation from a fracture should start the moment he enters the Accident and Emergency department. The nurse should be able to advise the patient how long he will have to wear the cast. Generally 6 weeks should be allowed for a Colles' fracture to unite, 8 weeks for a fracture of the humerus, 6 weeks for a fracture of the lateral malleolus and up to 14 weeks for a fracture of the tibial shaft.

Therefore, the patient can be given an estimate as to how long he will be immobile. Every encouragement should be given for him to maintain the function of his peripheral joints. The occupational therapist can assist, especially with elderly ladies, because of her ability to assess their competence in their domestic situation. If they are clearly unable to look after themselves, the medical social worker will arrange for a home help to call and assist with the household chores.

The patient who has sustained an industrial injury can frequently return to work at an early date. The doctor should notify the firm requesting that he returns to work as soon as possible, even if the limb is encased in a plaster cast. The waterproof thermoplastic materials are of special benefit when the patient returns to work while continuing treatment.

9

Eye injuries

A. H. DAVIES

Foreign bodies

Many small foreign bodies in the eye, such as dust, or eye-lashes, may be removed by the nursing staff. The doctor then only needs to check that everything is satisfactory.

Success depends upon:

(1) A good movable light.
(2) A steady patient who should lie down with his head on a small firm pillow, or sit either in a chair with a head rest or with his head against a wall. Support of the head is essential because many people involuntarily retreat when approached for an eye examination.
(3) The nurse should reassure the patient, stand back and then take a good general look at him and at both his eyes before she approaches closer to inspect his affected eye or touch his face. Although this principle is true for all patient examinations it is especially important when dealing with eyes, which are very sensitive organs.
(4) A systematic examination. The lower lid is pulled down by one finger on the skin below the lashes to expose the conjunctiva. The patient is told to look up, then to each side. The light is directed to illuminate the eye from different angles, sometimes disclosing a very small foreign body by producing or altering its shadow.

The upper lid may be everted to demonstrate its lining conjunctiva by rolling it upwards over a match, orange stick or probe (Figure 9.1a–c). In this maneuver the nurse grasps the eyelashes of the upper lid between her thumb (Figure 9.1a) and forefinger and tells the patient to look at his feet. Then, with her other hand, she holds the probe horizontally in the skin groove above the eye (Figure 9.1b), and with the hand holding the lashes she everts the lid over the probe. This exposes the conjunctiva lining the upper lid (Figure 9.1c), often revealing a previously hidden and adherent foreign body.

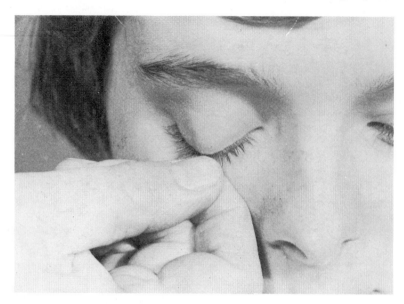

Figure 9.1a   Everting the upper lid. Pull down upper lid, hold lashes between finger and thumb

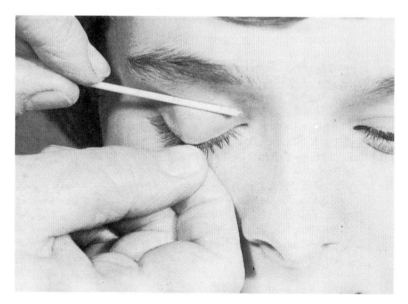

Figure 9.1b   Hold probe in groove above eye. Patient looks towards his feet

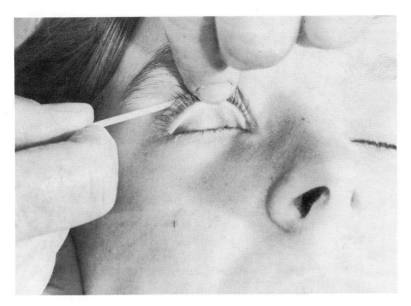

Figure 9.1c   Evert lid using probe as a lever, revealing conjunctiva lining upper
lid

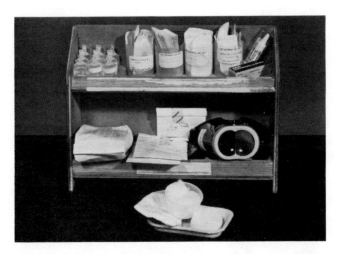

Figure 9.2   'Eye tray' for eye examination and treatment. Contains individual
squeezy ampules of sterile water or saline, individual dosage packs
or capsules of local anesthetic, fluorescein, sulfacetamide drops
and chloramphenical drops, tube of chloramphenical ointment,
sterile eye pads in packets, ophthalmic loupe

The conjunctiva of the globe above the cornea is not fully exposed during the latter maneuver; a better view is obtained if the patient looks down, as before, while the nurse lifts the lid up and away from the eye with one finger without turning the lid inside out.

The cornea is best inspected with the ophthalmic 'loupe' (Figure 9.2) which is simply a pair of goggles with high magnification. To locate a corneal foreign body while wearing the loupe the nurse asks the patient to move the eye slowly in all directions. As before, the adjustable light may also be moved about, to produce the shadowing effect of a foreign body.

REMOVAL OF A FOREIGN BODY

A foreign body located by the above examination may be carefully flicked off with the corner of a gauze swab or a well wrapped cotton swab.

If no foreign body is found, the eye is irrigated with water or normal saline, preferably from small plastic squeezy bottles each containing 10 ml single-use doses. These are safer to use than the old-fashioned glass ophthalmic irrigator with its inherent dangers of breakage and cross infection.

If the scratchiness or irritation remains after irrigation, she asks the doctor to examine the eye, because the foreign body may be adherent to or embedded in the cornea, or the soreness may have some other cause.

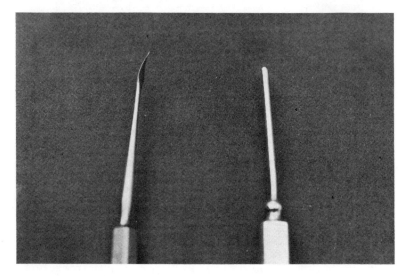

Figure 9.3   Needle and spud. left: sharp pointed eye 'needle', right: round sided eye 'spud'

The doctor will need the loupe and the light, and also require an eye spud and an eye needle. These are probe-like instruments with either a flattened round end (spud) or a flattened but pointed end (needle) (Figure 9.3). They should be sterilized between each patient's use, either by autoclaving or by storage in hexachlorophane in spirit or instrument chloroxylenol. The nurse must be careful to rinse the instrument in sterile water before use if the latter method is employed.

Local analgesia
Local analgesia is necessary for removal of an adherent corneal foreign body. Amethocaine hydrochloride (tetracaine) 0.5% solution, is a popular agent which is available in individual dose ampoules. Two or three drops are instilled inside the lower lid and the eye is closed. Within 2 or 3 minutes the cornea and conjunctiva become analgesic and remain so for 15–20 minutes.

Protective eye pads
For the following 2–3 hours there will be a partial analgesia during which time the eye must be covered to protect it from other minute foreign bodies. Normally these would be cleared by a reactive increase in tear formation or by the blink mechanism.

A sterile cotton wool and gauze pad is lightly applied and kept in place with a non-allergic adhesive tape. The patient should be informed of the reason for wearing the pad and be told when to remove it. He should also be advised to avoid matches or cigarette lighters near the face while wearing a pad otherwise they may set both pad and tape on fire. Plastic eye shields should not be worn as they tend to retain moisture and warmth and thus encourage growth of pathological organisms. If long term protection of the eye is required the patient is advised to wear a pair of dark glasses.

CORNEAL ABRASIONS, LACERATIONS AND ULCERS
Removal of an embedded corneal foreign body damages the surface of the cornea causing an abrasion or ulcer. Even if a foreign body has not been located but the patient complains of the sensation of 'something still there', there may be an abrasion from a previously dislodged foreign body or a corneal ulcer from some other cause. However, corneal injury may not be apparent until stained by the dye fluorescein, which is available in small, individual dose ampoules. One drop is usually sufficient as it spreads very quickly in the tears. Fluorescein shows up any break in the surface of the cornea as a bright orange-green colour. After using fluorescein the eye and eyelids should be rinsed with sterile water or the patient may leave the department with a distinctive orange eye!

Corneal ulcers and abrasions are usually treated in the first instance by:

(1) Rest – the eye is covered with an eye pad.
(2) A mydriatic agent (atropine or homatropine ointment or drops) to dilate the pupil and further rest the eye.
(3) A local antibiotic such as chloramphenicol or sulphacetamide (sulfacetamide) ointment or drops, applied or instilled three or four times a day.

Any corneal injury which does not heal within a week on this regimen must be referred to the ophthalmologist.

Serious eye injuries

The Accident and Emergency doctor and nurse must be able to recognize the more serious eye injuries which need prompt attention from an ophthalmologist.

Contusion of the globe from direct blows from a tennis ball etc., laceration of the globe and a penetrating injury must all be treated urgently.

In addition to the case history the following appearances indicate serious injury:

(1) Bleeding or distortion of the eye.
(2) A widely dilated or irregular shaped pupil (Figure 9.4)
(3) Blood in the anterior chamber (between the cornea and the iris), called a hyphema, is often seen as a dark fluid level when the patient is vertical (Figure 9.5).

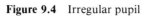

Figure 9.4 Irregular pupil   **Figure 9.5** Hyphema

The patient should be laid down on a couch or trolley (gurney) immediately on arrival in the department. This lowers the intra-ocular pressure by relaxing the patient and reducing the movement of the head. A sterile pad is applied to the eye and further examination is left to the doctor. If a penetrating foreign body is suspected an X-ray is taken, and a systemic antibiotic is usually prescribed. The patient must remain lying down whilst waiting for and during transfer to the X-ray department or for admission to the ward.

Non-traumatic conditions

Occasionally a patient attends the Accident and Emergency department following the sudden onset of an acutely painful eye condition because he thinks that there may be a foreign body present.

Acute conjunctivitis, iritis, irido-cyclitis, and acute glaucoma, are all conditions which may arise suddenly with pain and inflammation. If the nurse sees a patient with a very red, inflamed and painful eye condition, it is unwise to start examining it herself; she should wait for the doctor to differentiate between a simple foreign body and a non-traumatic condition. If the doctor diagnoses conjunctivitis, he prescribes a local antibiotic ointment or drops. If it is a more serious condition he will probably not start any definitive treatment, but refer the patient urgently to the ophthalmologist.

10

Ear, nose and throat, and facio-maxillary injuries

A. H. DAVIES

Injury or emergency conditions involving the mouth, ears, nose or throat are often treated in separate specialist departments but initially many patients attend the Accident and Emergency department, and the nurse must therefore be able to render suitable treatment.

Foreign bodies

Small children from toddlers to early school age are frequently brought to hospital after pushing small objects into various bodily orifices. The mouth, nose and ears are conveniently available to receive such things as peas, chalk, beads, paper clips, sweets, pen nibs and even open safety pins.

Occasionally older children, even into their early teens, are involved, but usually the adults who attend with this complaint are mentally subnormal.

NOSE

Sometimes a recently inserted foreign body can clearly be seen in the nostril. It is tempting for the nurse to try and retrieve it quickly before it disappears. However, this is unwise because the attempt may be unsuccessful and may push in the foreign body further. What is more, a crying, struggling child may inhale it, thus obstructing the larynx or trachea.

Removal of a foreign body from the nostril requires patience and a calm unhurried approach. As when examining the eye, a good light, a stable position for the patient and a selection of instruments are necessary for success (see Figure 10.3).

The child is less likely to cry if sat up. A good firm hold on a small child is obtained by sitting it on the lap of the parent or nurse who holds the arms with one hand, and its head against her chest with the other (Figure 10.1). The child is prevented from kicking by securing its legs firmly between the adult's knees. This hold should not be adopted until the doctor, the light and the instruments are ready. If the child is uncontrollable then the risk of him crying and struggling has to be taken; he is wrapped up firmly in a blanket (Figure 10.2) and is examined lying on his side.

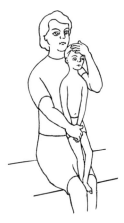

Figure 10.1 Position for holding small child for examination of eyes, ears, nose, mouth or throat

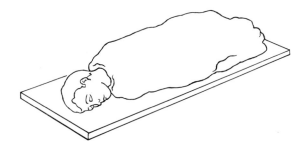

Figure 10.2 Small child, wrapped in blanket with head lower than chest, ready for stomach lavage

With the older child it is worth while talking to him and explaining what is being done and why. He may be persuaded to try to blow out the foreign body, using one finger (his or the nurse's) to occlude the other nostril. However, the nurse must be quite sure the child knows that he is to blow and not to sniff, as most younger children sniff vigorously when asked to blow their nose.

If blowing the nose does not succeed, the doctor tries to hook the foreign body down the nostril. This procedure requires a nostril dilator, a long narrow shafted Volkmann's spoon, and a hook with a sharp point. Long narrow toothed or clawed forceps are sometimes used to grasp a soft foreign body such as a piece of chalk or a peanut. Plain forceps are dangerous because they slide off most foreign bodies and may shoot them further up the nose.

If the foreign body has been present for more than 24 hours the mucosal lining of the nostril produces a copious green discharge which obscures the view. The doctor will then probably decide not to proceed if he cannot see the object, but refer the child to the Ear, Nose and Throat (ENT) department.

After simple removal of a foreign body no further treatment or review is necessary.

EARS

Again, a good light and the child in a stable position are necessary. Some doctors are adept at using a head mirror, which reflects a narrow beam of light exactly where it is wanted. Others prefer an auriscope with a wide speculum.

Most foreign bodies come out of the ear during gentle syringing with lukewarm water or normal saline except the dried pea which, in the presence of water, swells and becomes further impacted. Occasionally an object can be easily grasped or eased out with the hook used for the removal of nasal foreign bodies.

INHALED FOREIGN BODIES

These are much more worrying, potentially life threatening and most often involve children and old people. The variety of foreign bodies involved is similar to that found in the nose or ear (p. 84), with the addition of half-chewed food such as meat.

The patient may arrive distressed and gasping for breath, or he may be breathing quietly. He may be 'rattling' or 'grunting', sometimes cyanosed (p. 162) and in desperate need of help.

If the situation appears urgent to the receiving nurse in that she finds a panicstricken, dyspneic, and cyanosed patient, she may have to act promptly to save life before the doctor arrives.

A *small child* or baby should be held upside down by the legs and jolted up and down. This makes it cry, cough or vomit, and hopefully, combined with the influence of gravity, causes the ejection of the foreign body and clears the airway.

An *older child* may be too big for this procedure to be practical. He is then held face down over the knees of the nurse who, sitting on a firm seat with the child's head and chest hanging down, presses or thumps the back of his chest.

An *adult* is obviously too large for the above procedures. The nurse therefore approaches him from behind and makes a quick, sharp grab around the patient's upper abdomen. This produces a sudden forceful expiration, and occasionally dislodges and ejects the foreign body.

If such maneuvers do not relieve the situation they should not be repeated more than once or twice: the patient should be laid, sloping head down, on a trolley (gurney) in the three-quarters prone position. The nurse then administers oxygen by face mask or by nasal catheter whilst her colleague prepares a tray for an immediate laryngoscopy, bronchoscopy and tracheostomy. At least one sterile emergency tracheostomy pack should always be available in the resuscitation area and the nurse must be familiar with its contents.

If the Emergency doctor is inexperienced and unwilling to attempt a tracheostomy, a large bore needle, or a trocar and cannula can produce some relief. The needle is introduced in the midline of the neck through the crico-thyroid membrane or at a lower level just below the first ring of the trachea. Although this provides only a very small airway it may enable the patient to survive until a more experienced general surgical or ENT specialist arrives.

If the patient is neither distressed nor dyspneic on admission there is no urgency and all that is required is a nurse to talk to the patient, reassure him, and sit him down in a chair, while awaiting his routine turn to be examined by the doctor. X-ray of the throat, neck, and chest may confirm the presence of a foreign body or demonstrate its effects as collapsed areas (atelectasis) in the lung fields whereupon bronchoscopy or laryngoscopy will be essential.

SWALLOWED FOREIGN BODIES

Most swallowed foreign bodies pass down into the stomach and cause no problems. The patient (or the parents if the patient is a child) only needs reassuring by the nurse and doctor that trouble is unlikely to arise. Many patients or parents expect or even demand an X-ray examination, which is only helpful if the object is of bone or metal, because plastic, wood and some glass are not radio-opaque. Having established that a foreign body has been swallowed, and unlikely to do harm, the parents must be instructed to inspect the child's stools (using a 'potty' for a while) until the object appears. The child should be brought back for re-examination if he develops pain or vomiting, or if the object is not discharged within 7 days.

Occasionally sharp objects, such as fish or chicken bones, lodge in a tonsil or in the posterior pharyngeal wall from which they are easily removed by the doctor if they are visible and the patient is co-operative. Frequently, the sensation that 'something is there' persists when in fact there is only an abrasion, the foreign body having passed down the esophagus into the stomach. If a sharp object, such as an open safety pin, does lodge at the lower end of the esophagus then the patient needs admitting for esophagoscopy.

Injuries
Patients with minor bruises of the face, nose, cheeks or chin may require radiological examination to exclude fracture. Usually all they need is reassurance.

FRACTURED NOSE
This injury is very common. The nose is swollen and bruised and may be flattened or deflected to one side. There is usually bleeding fron one or both nostrils but rarely enough to warrant the insertion of a nasal pack. Most specialists before correcting the deformity prefer to assess it first, usually after the swelling has gone down, but within 5–10 days of the accident.

More serious injuries and facial fractures may give rise to serious airway problems.

DEPRESSED AND COMPOUND FRACTURES
Fractures of the middle and lower thirds of the face cause difficulty in maintaining the airway, and the patient may have to lie with his head over the end or side of the trolley or even supported by the nurse's hands or arms, so that the soft tissues fall forwards due to gravity and relieve some of the obstruction. If these patients are conscious they are very distressed and require considerable physical support and encouragement, until an anesthetist and a facio-maxillary surgeon arrive to introduce an endotracheal tube or perform a tracheostomy.

Epistaxis
Spontaneous bleeding from the nose may occur at any age. The patient sometimes walks in, clutching a bloody rag to his face and is often worried and distressed if the bleeding has been going on for some time.

The best position for the patient to adopt is to sit up on a trolley or couch, reclining comfortably against the back rest. Relaxation is essential because tension and fuss tend to prolong the bleeding. Swallowed blood irritates the stomach and causes vomiting, and a bowl should be provided in case the patient wants to spit or vomit.

The patient is then told to sit up and 'pinch' his own nose, including all the soft part below the nasal bones, between his finger and thumb and to breathe through his mouth. This pressure stops most bleeding if steadily maintained for 5 or more minutes.

However, the doctor will still wish to examine the patient to confirm that the bleeding has stopped and ensure that blood is not quietly trickling down the back of the throat. He will also assess whether the patient is shocked from blood loss and try to discover any underlying cause of the hemorrhage. If hypertension is responsible then the elderly patient may be comforted by being told that the nose bleed is a safety valve and nature's own way of helping to relieve the condition. However, the bleeding must be stopped or the patient may become exsanguinated.

If simple measures do not arrest the hemorrhage then the nose probably needs to be packed. Although the nurse is sometimes asked to insert the pack the doctor usually prefers to do it himself.

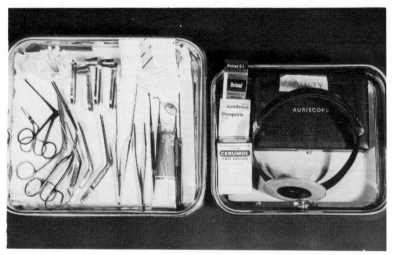

Figure 10.3 ENT examination trays containing cottonwool buds, nasal specula, lubricating jelly for nasal pack, ear drops, auriscope, head mirror, sterile pack of ribbon gauze for nasal packs

Requirements (Figure 10.3)

  (1) A good light
  (2) Nasal specula
  (3) 0.5 cm (¼ in) ribbon gauze in a roll, 2–3 m long, and scissors to cut the appropriate length.
  (4) Lubricating jelly.
  (5) Small gallipot to soak the gauze in the jelly.
  (6) Long narrow ended forceps to hold and insert the gauze.
  (7) Gauze swabs (pads) and water for cleaning.
  (8) Adhesive tape to keep the pack in place.

Before packing is started the doctor may order a sedative such as diazepam which is given intramuscularly because oral medication is likely to be vomited. Morphine is an alternative choice.

After the pack is inserted the patient should be left to relax, with a bowl and a supply of swabs. He should be checked every 15 mins to make sure his pulse and colour are satisfactory.

When the bleeding has stopped for more than an hour the patient is allowed to leave, provided he has someone at home and suitable transport to take him there. He is told to rest and to return 1–2 days later for the removal of the pack.

If the bleeding continues or recurs the patient is referred to the Ear, Nose and Throat (ENT) department for cauterization of the bleeding area. Occasionally, if the bleeding originates further back in the nose in a position inaccessible to cauterization, a special 'balloon' catheter is introduced into the nostril and inflated so that it applies pressure to the bleeding point.

Bleeding tooth socket
Occasionally after tooth extraction the socket continues to bleed slightly. This may not bother the patient much during the day, but towards evening and night time it may increase a little, he notices it more, or he is worried that it will increase later. Consequently, late evening is the commonest time for patients with post-extraction hemorrhage to present themselves in the Accident and Emergency department.

Treatment follows that which is generally applied to any other hemorrhage namely elevation, rest, reassurance, and local pressure. As in the treatment of epistaxis (p. 88) the patient is sat up on a trolley or couch supported by the back rest so that he can relax with his head elevated. The pulse and blood pressure are taken and recorded. A water-proof cape or bib around the neck helps to protect the patient's clothes because he may dribble bloodstained saliva during the treatment.

The nurse then applies pressure by inserting a small tight roll of gauze between the teeth adjacent to the socket and projecting above them (Figure 10.4).

The patient is then told to bite hard, so that the pack is forced down onto the bleeding area. This procedure stops most bleeding from sockets if maintained for 10 or more minutes.

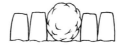

Figure 10.4   Dental pack

However, if the bleeding persists, the doctor examines the socket, removes any clot or debris and inserts an adrenaline (epinephrine) soaked pack (1 in 10 000 solution) or one made of hemostatic absorbable foam or gauze. A fresh dry gauze pack is also inserted and the patient instructed to bite hard as before.

If the patient is distressed the doctor may prescribe diazepam or morphia as in the treatment of epistaxis. Very rarely a patient may bleed enough to require transfusion with a plasma expander (p. 136), plasma or blood, followed by admission to the ward for further observation. If the bleeding persists the socket may have to be sutured with silk or synthetic suture on an atraumatic three-quarter circle cutting needle.

'Secondary' hemorrhage, which occurs several days after extraction and is due to infection, is similarly treated but with the addition of an antibiotic.

Toothache

This is another common evening or weekend complaint, when the patient presents in the Emergency department because he cannot contact his own dentist for treatment or advice. The toothache sufferer usually tries to obtain relief with the common analgesic tablets, aspirin, paracetamol (acetaminophen), codeine or proprietary mixtures of these.

The doctor requires a good light and a sterile metal or disposable wooden spatula. If infection is present he prescribes an antibiotic and releases the pus from any fluctuating abscess through a small incision in the gum, a procedure which often gives immediate pain relief.

It may be unnecessary to give an anesthetic if the incision is made confidently and quickly with a sharp pointed scalpel. In the nervous patient analgesia is achieved by means of either a local analgesic spray or a gauze swab soaked in 2–3 ml of 1% plain lignocaine (lidocaine) applied adjacent to the affected gums for a few minutes before incision.

Most doctors do not attempt to remove a carious tooth because they are insufficiently trained in the technique of extraction and usually there are no suitable instruments available in the department. However, if the offending tooth has a hollow cavity it can be packed with a small pledgelet of cotton wool (cotton) which has been soaked in oil of cloves. This traditional household remedy sometimes gives some relief because it has a mild analgesic effect on an exposed nerve and when combined with analgesic tablets may pacify the patient until he can contact a dentist.

Narcotics such as morphia and pethidine are rarely used because of the dangers of addiction.

11

Self-inflicted injuries

A. H. DAVIES

Self-inflicted injuries are very common and present many special problems to the nursing staff of the Accident and Emergency department.

Patients who have taken an overdose of a poisonous substance form the greatest proportion of self-inflicted injuries; 20–30 years ago deliberate self-administration of an overdose was rare but usually constituted a serious suicidal attempt which succeeded because treatment was ineffective.

The true suicide attempt takes a massive overdose of something that is likely to be fatal. He then hides himself away so that he remains undiscovered until it is too late to save his life.

In recent years, the incidence of self-poisoning has increased considerably. Many of these people are in effect trying to say to their relatives, spouses or lovers such things as 'Help' – 'Please notice me', 'I am really miserable' or 'Sorry' and sometimes 'Perhaps I'll die and then you'll be sorry'. Impulsively they take whatever is to hand, especially the unused tablets and medicines that have accumulated at home over the years, but in a quantity usually insufficient to be lethal. Also, they ensure that someone knows about their action, often immediately after swallowing the last pill.

When an overdose patient arrives in hospital he is usually in a very vulnerable emotional state and a sympathetic nurse can often obtain the whole sad story including the type and quantity of drug taken and when it was swallowed long before a psychiatrist arrives to assess his mental condition.

Nursing management
However irritating the nurse finds the bogus suicide, she should always regard every patient as being a true suicide attempt.

A stomach washout should never be started before the doctor arrives, because this procedure may be ineffective if the overdose has been taken more than 4 hours previously. Furthermore, the presence of an anesthetist is essential in dealing with the comatose or semicomatose patient (p. 178) to prevent the inhalation of washout fluid or stomach contents.

Refusal to accept a stomach washout must be respected, otherwise the nursing staff may be accused of assault when the patient has recovered. It is always unwise and dangerous to try to hold down or wrestle with someone in order to pass a gastric tube.

The nurse should ensure that the patient who is discharged has a home or other suitable accommodation and also has someone there to help him in his troubles, because the majority need ordinary sympathetic and understanding human contact rather than psychiatric help or medical skill. The nurse often has to solve this type of problem if no social worker is available.

The drunk
Every Accident and Emergency department has its share of well known chronic alcoholics. Sometimes such an inidividual is brought in having been found collapsed on the street or may have fallen, suffering minor injuries such as scalp lacerations, a nasal fracture, split lips, or bruised and grazed limbs. The drunk usually falls over limply, saving himself from more serious injuries. Occasionally, however, he may injure himself more severely but because he is 'anesthetized' by the alcohol he complains little about his injuries (p. 212). Consequently, although it is often an unpleasant and difficult task, the drunk should always be undressed and fully examined. It is not unusual for a cheerful but fully conscious drunk to be sent to the X-ray department and return the worse for wear, lapsing into unconsciousness because the nurse has not discovered a bottle, concealed in a pocket of his usually voluminous coat, the contents of which he has quietly enjoyed whilst awaiting treatment. It must also be remembered that the incoordination of intoxication may cause the drunk to tip up a wheelchair or climb and fall out of even a cot-sided trolley (gurney) and so cause himself further damage.

To summarize:

(1) The drunk must never be trusted.
(2) The drunk should not be left alone.
(3) Serious injury must not be missed.
(4) The drunk must not be discharged home or into the custody of the police whilst still drowsy or incoordinate, and certainly not when unconscious in case there is an additional medical cause for his condition.

Ideally, every department should have a 'Safe' room with mattresses on the floor to enable such patients to sleep it off.

Drug abuse
Although drug abuse affects all ages and most branches of society, it is especially common in the young and the dropout. They often have a culture and language of their own and refer to their drugs by a variety of colloquial names. Addiction can occur with either soft drugs (cannabis) hallucinators (lysergic acid – LSD) and hard drugs (morphia and diamorphine – heroin). Although these patients present in different ways, they usually fall into three main categories:

(1) The patient is brought to the hospital, by the police or by friends, following a massive overdose of the drug to which he is addicted.
(2) The patient has taken a drug whose effects on him are unfamiliar and he has become frightened.
(3) After taking a hallucinatory drug he may sustain injury when performing some dangerous action e.g., jumping off a bridge or walking in front of a bus, because in this unreal state of consciousness he was unappreciative of the danger or he considered it desirable.
(4) He is unable to obtain his next 'fix' and is hoping to obtain it from the hospital. Such patients create difficulties for the nursing staff, they tend to wander about the department looking for drugs or needles and syringes and may become a nuisance and abusive. They may even start to develop withdrawal symptoms.

The Accident and Emergency nurse should not waste time and effort trying to reform and 'dry out' these addicts. It is a long and thankless task and is best left to people who are trained and dedicated to the work. A psychiatric social worker may be helpful and in some areas there is a drug-abuse center to which the patients may be referred for help if that is what they want.

Self-inflicted physical injuries
Patients who attempt to cut their wrists or throat (Figure 11.1a and b), stab or shoot themselves, or inflict other traumatic injuries are easier to deal with because there is something immediately obvious to be done in the way of treatment. These are usually people who really mean to commit suicide, but as their knowledge of anatomy is frequently poor

they often miss wounding the vital parts and simply end up in a bloody mess but still alive.

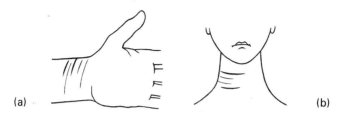

(a)   (b)

Figure 11.1   Tentative lacerations of wrist and neck to different depths
　　　　　　(a)   Left wrist lacerations are usually self-inflicted if the patient is right-handed
　　　　　　(b)   Right-sided neck lacerations are usually self-inflicted if the patient is left-handed

IMMEDIATE TREATMENT

(1)   Quickly assess the general condition of the patient and send for help if necessary.
(2)   If unconscious, attend to the airway.
(3)   If there is severe bleeding, identify its site of origin, cover with sterile swabs or towels, apply pressure and elevate (if practicable) the bleeding part (p. 37).
(4)   If shocked, lay the patient down, lift the foot of the trolley (gurney) and prepare an intravenous infusion.
(5)   There may be injury to the respiratory tract due to a stab wound in the chest or a self-administered tracheostomy; the latter sometimes results if the patient tries to cut his throat with the chin elevated, thus bringing the trachea forwards so that it is easily injured. However, the main blood vessels are missed because they tend to slide backwards. Tracheal injury usually produces a sucking sound with respiratory embarrassment until the wound is covered. This should be done first with a sterile cloth, followed by something fairly airtight such as plastic sheeting which is then secured by adhesive strapping. The patient is usually more comfortable and can breathe more easily if sat up, and this position should be adopted unless he is in a state of shock. Oxygen should always be given. The patient must always be fully undressed to enable the doctor to look for other injuries.
(6)   The patient, his friends and relatives are asked if he has done anything else to speed his death such as taking an overdose.

Carbon monoxide poisoning

The carbon monoxide present in car exhaust fumes is rapid in its effects provided that it is inhaled in an enclosed space. Sometimes the victim takes elaborate precautions to shut and seal all windows and ventilators of the car, and by means of a tube leads the carbon monoxide from the exhaust into the car's interior.

DIAGNOSIS OF CARBON MONOXIDE POISONING

Appearance

The appearance of a person poisoned by carbon monoxide is deceptive, because although he is usually unconscious he is not cyanosed. The pinkness of his skin is due to the bright red colouration produced by the formation of carboxyhemoglobin, i.e. when the inhaled carbon monoxide combines with hemoglobin. Because hemoglobin has a greater affinity for the carbon monoxide than it has for oxygen the patient suffers from oxygen lack even if the carbon monoxide inhaled is of low concentration.

Respiration

The depth of respiration is shallow and eventually the patient becomes apnoeic.

Emergency treatment

Restore and maintain the airway by supporting the chin, and insert an oral airway (p. 168). Administer oxygen if necessary by intermittent positive pressure ventilation (IPPV – p. 221) with an Ambu resuscitation bag (p. 224).

When adequate help is available the patient is undressed completely to exclude other injuries and to ensure there is no other cause for the unconsciousness such as a cerebrovascular accident. Blood is sent for analysis because the patient may also have taken a drug overdose to ensure his demise.

Drowning

Drowning is occasionally used as a method of suicide by the older patient who is brought into hospital cold, wet and apparently dead. Diagnosis of death on clinical grounds in a hypothermic patient is difficult or impossible and so resuscitation is started and continued until electrocardiography proves conclusively that the patient is dead. The nurse lowers the head of the trolley (gurney) to allow gravitational drainage of fluid from the mouth, nose and lungs, and aspirates water, mucus, vomit etc. by means of a suction apparatus.

She gives oxygen by IPPV and makes arrangements for the electrical activity of the heart to be recorded using an ECG (EKG). The cardiac arrest team is alerted and preparations are made to perform external cardiac massage (p. 261).

When some sort of order has been established the wet, cold clothes are removed from the patient who is then covered with warm, dry blankets to prevent further heat loss.

Other suicides

Jumping off a bridge, or stepping in front of a bus or train, are fortunately uncommon methods of suicide, but naturally produce severe multiple injuries. The patient is usually shocked, bleeding and unconscious. Treatment is similar to that involving the victim of a road traffic accident as discussed in chapter 3.

12

Infections

V. W. BURTON

Although they are not strictly either 'accidents' or 'emergencies' many cases of sepsis are dealt with in most Accident and Emergency departments. Many general practitioners have neither the time nor the facilities for incision of abscesses, particularly if a general anaesthetic is required and, if the patients are referred to the General Surgical department, they may have to wait for an out-patient appointment.

Hand infections

ACUTE PARONYCHIA

This is an infection of the nail fold and is the most common infection encountered in the hand, particularly in housewives who frequently immerse their hands in detergent. The infection starts at the margin of the nail; pain, swelling and local erythema develop (Figure 12.1). At this stage of infection many resolve completely without the formation of pus if the patient is given antibiotics and the digit is protected from water. If the infection progresses, subcuticular pus forms at the lateral margin of the nail which needs evacuating in the minor operating theatre of the Accident and Emergency department.

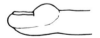

Figure 12.1   Paronychia

The nurse arranges a trolley (cart) with syringes, needles and 1% lignocaine (lidocaine) solution for analgesia under a ring block (p. 17). Once analgesia is complete the doctor drains the collection of pus by making a small incision with a number 15 scalpel blade over the corner of the nail.

Involvement of the proximal half of the nail with pus oozing from the nail fold necessitates removal of the base of the nail. After drainage the cavity is packed with antibiotic impregnated vaseline tulle and the patient told to attend for regular dressings.

BOILS AND CARBUNCLES
These are commonly found on the back of the hand where the skin is loose. They are due to a staphylococcal infection of hair follicles. They are more common in diabetic patients and the spontaneous appearance of boils should alert the medical and nursing staff to the possible diagnosis of diabetes. Therefore, as a routine precaution a specimen of urine should be obtained from the patient and tested for sugar.

Initially the hand is elevated in a sling, an antibiotic given such as penicillin, provided there is no history of sensitivity, and the boil is regularly dressed. If the lesion 'points' and pus is visible the subcuticular abscess is de-roofed with sharp scissors and the cavity cleaned with antiseptic solution before being lightly packed with an antibiotic impregnated tulle. The discharge from the septic area may be encouraged by the use of a magnesium sulphate paste dressing but this is quite useless if the skin is still intact.

PALMAR SPACE INFECTION
In the hand there are several potential spaces all of which may be the seat of infection after a penetrating wound. The skin is thick and firmly anchored on the palm of the hand so deep infection may present with swelling under the loose skin over the *dorsum* of the hand. As the tissue tension in the palm of the hand increases with the appearance of pus, pain becomes more severe and the patient becomes toxic with a high fever. Local tenderness and swelling are now evident in the palm of the hand. The spread of infection through the lymphatics in the arm leads to lymphangitis and lymphadenitis. Lymphangitis is recognized by an appearance of red streaks in the forearm in the line of the lymphatic vessels, while lymphadenitis results in tender enlargement of the axillary lymph nodes which drain the infected lymph from the hand.

A small localized superficial abscess can be completely drained in the Accident and Emergency department. If there is involvement of the deep tissues of the palm the patient is admitted to a ward for systemic antibiotic treatment, elevation of the limb and probable clearance of the abscess cavity under general anesthesia with the aid of a tourniquet, which allows the surgeon to identify the important peripheral nerves when evacuating the pus.

PULP SPACE INFECTION
The soft tissues of the end finger segment may become infected by a penetrating injury such as that caused by a rose thorn. If the infection is

treated inadequately the tissue tension rises, and the nutrient arteries of the terminal phalanx become thrombosed with the development of osteomyelitis (inflammation of the bone), and eventual sequestration (death and separation) of the terminal phalanx. Therefore, diagnosis and adequate treatment are important.

The nurse should suspect the presence of a pulp space infection following a penetrating injury if the patient complains of a throbbing pain at the finger tip which may be swollen and tender (Figure 12.2). If there is no sign of pus the hand should be elevated in a sling and antibiotics prescribed. If pus is visible, drainage is indicated.

Figure 12.2   Pulp space infection

A ring block or preferably a general anesthetic is administered in the minor operating theatre and the abscess opened using a number 15 scalpel blade. A specimen of pus is sent to the laboratory for culture and sensitivity testing. The cavity is loosely packed with either fucidin tulle or sofra tulle, and the patient told to attend for regular dressings until wound healing is complete. The development of a sinus with a persistent discharge suggests bone death with the formation of a sequestrum. The patient then needs referral for a specialist opinion.

Other infections
Patients suffering from infective lesions elsewhere, such as axillary or inguinal abscesses, infected sebaceous cysts or infection arising from bites, may attend the Accident and Emergency department or be referred there by their own physicians.

The principles of treatment are always the same; if pus is not evident, local rest perhaps with splintage, elevation if possible and appropriate antibiotics are usually all that is required. If pus accumulates, incision under local analgesia or general anesthesia is indicated, followed by regular dressings until wound healing is complete. A specimen of pus should always be sent to the bacteriological laboratory with a request for culture and sensitivity testing. Many of the abscesses dealt with in the Accident and Emergency department are due to *Staphylococcus aureus* but occasionally other bacteria such as the tubercle bacillus may be implicated.

Breast abscess

Breast abscesses occur most frequently in lactating women. Should the abscess require incising, the dressing may be conveniently held in place using the patient's own cotton maternity or nursing brassière. The patient must be advised whether or not to continue with breast feeding. Usually she is told to continue feeding with the normal breast but to empty the infected breast by means of a pump and discard the milk even though it is not usually contaminated with bacteria.

Perineal and vulval abscesses

As much hair as possible should be shaved off prior to incision as this simplifies the subsequent dressings.

The position of the patient prior to incision of the abscess is discussed with the surgeon and anesthetist. The patient may lie on either side or is supported in the lithotomy position.

The dressings are held in place with the traditional cotton bandage, which is a large maternity sanitary towel with tape or elastic at the waist. Alternatively, an elasticated tubular bandage may be cut into the shape of a pair of shorts.

Ingrowing toenail

This condition usually affects the great toe and is sometimes caused or aggravated by cutting the nail short and wearing tight shoes. Infection similar to a paronychia in the finger develops at the side of the nail which may be abnormally thick.

Occasionally, early treatment with local antiseptic dressings and avoiding excessive trimming of the lateral margins of the nail is effective. However, if the infection has become chronic it will not resolve until the lateral margin of the nail is removed, to allow the drainage of any deep seated pus.

Resection of the lateral nail margin is performed under infiltration analgesia with a 1% solution of lignocaine, using a similar technique to that described for establishing a finger ring block (p. 17).

The doctor requires a tissue forceps, e.g. a pair of Kocher's, a small scalpel holder with a number 15 blade and a pair of sharp scissors.

After removal of the nail portion, a vaseline tulle dressing impregnated with antibiotic is applied, and the patient told to attend for dressings on alternate days until the nail bed has healed and no evidence of infection remains.

The nurse should teach the patient the correct method of nail cutting, i.e. cutting the nail transversely and avoiding any trimming of the nail edges.

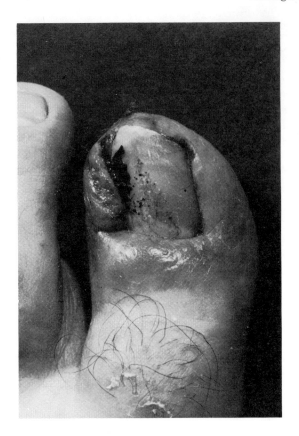

Figure 12.3a   Chronic septic ingrowing toenail. Note granulations. Both sides
have been cut short, down into corners, leaving a hidden spike
buried in the soft tissue at the side

Figure 12.3b   The removed ingrowing toenail, shown in Figure 12.3(a). Note
spike which acts as a foreign body

The patient is asked to wash his feet regularly, paying particular attention to the area around the nail, removing all dirt and dead skin. He is also advised to avoid wearing tight shoes.

Excision of the nail along with the nail bed is indicated should an ingrowing toenail recur.

13

Local analgesia

J. E. PRING

Local analgesics are used for many of the procedures carried out in the Accident and Emergency department. The selective use of nerve blocks can supplement general anesthesia, contribute towards intra-operative analgesia, and make the initial post-operative period more comfortable. Such a technique is adopted when a digital nerve block and removal of a toenail are performed under general anesthesia.

Advantages of local analgesia

PERSONAL CHOICE

Some patients are afraid to have a general anesthetic, and prefer to submit to local analgesia.

LACK OF HANGOVER

Some of the procedures carried out are of a relatively minor nature, e.g. incision of a paronychia, and do not require hospital admission. Local analgesia allows the patient to leave the hospital as soon as the operation is over, without having to recover from the hangover effects of general anesthesia. His early discharge saves bed space in the department, and spares the nurse, who would be delegated to look after him, for other duties.

Premedication is not essential, nor is it always desirable, because many of the narcotics and tranquillizers used in premedication have effects lasting much longer than the actual operative procedure. These vary according to the response of the individual, and include drowsiness, inability to appreciate or remember any instructions he is given, a lack of responsibility, incomplete awareness of his surroundings and irrational behaviour. Owing to the effects of tranquillizers he may faithfully promise not to drive home, yet be seen 5 minutes later at the wheel of his car. The consequent dangers of being involved in a road accident are obvious.

FREEDOM FROM SICKNESS

Other less dangerous but unpleasant effects due to drugs are avoided if premedication is omitted. For example, atropine causes a dry mouth, and opiates such as morphine may produce nausea and vomiting. On the other hand, drugs are sometimes blamed for producing these effects when in actual fact they are due to apprehension and fear. Nevertheless, many anesthetists do use intravenous sedative or tranquillizing drugs in association with a local analgesic.

REDUCED DANGERS OF THE FULL STOMACH

The patient may be totally unprepared for a general anesthetic, and may have to wait several hours before general anesthesia is considered safe. The major risk associated with general anesthesia is that of the full stomach, containing food, or fluid such as alcohol or the annoying 'cup of tea he had whilst waiting for the ambulance to arrive'. The full stomach is particularly dangerous under anesthesia, if active vomiting or passive reflux or regurgitation occurs (p. 178), because of the danger of stomach contents entering the pharynx, with overspill into the trachea and lungs. Massive aspiration results in the patient literally drowning, whilst lesser degrees of aspiration can cause an aspiration pneumonitis, with bronchospasm, cyanosis, and hypoxia (p. 163).

The usual policy is to wait 4 hours from the last intake of food or drink, and assume that the stomach is empty. However, this does not always solve the problem because fear, pain, and shock may delay gastric emptying. Accordingly, the anesthetist may prefer to use local analgesia rather than risk the patient vomiting whilst asleep, even though the patient has had nothing by mouth for several hours.

To ensure complete safety, if general anesthesia is essential, a less urgent procedure may have to be delayed for up to 12 hours, especially if the accident occurs soon after a large meal or the intake of large volumes of alcoholic drink.

Local analgesia is more time-consuming to administer and complete success is not as easy to achieve compared with general anesthesia but the risks, albeit small, of the latter are avoided.

LACK OF IMMEDIATE FACILITIES FOR GENERAL ANESTHESIA

At times, the general condition of the patient is a contraindication to general anesthesia, or facilities for skilled anesthesia are not readily available because the anesthetist has a number of more urgent cases waiting. If a local analgesic technique is used, the patient does not have to return home, continue fasting, and then make another journey to the hospital.

DOES THE NURSE INFLUENCE THE CHOICE OF ANESTHESIA?

The Accident and Emergency nurse often gives valuable guidance to the doctor because she has greater opportunity of watching the patient and either acquires or is given information which might influence treatment. For example, she may discover that the patient has a history of heart disease, previous myocardial infarction, angina, high blood pressure, respiratory disease or diabetes. Her routine attention in getting him ready for examination by the doctor may disclose the presence of swollen ankles, breathlessness, or the unusual aroma of his breath due to alcohol or diabetes. Recording his temperature, pulse, blood pressure and respiratory rate may provide other evidence of disease. Such findings by the nurse may influence or even decide that local analgesia is the safest choice.

AVOIDANCE OF REACTIONS TO INTRAVENOUS AGENTS USED IN GENERAL ANESTHESIA

Adverse reactions such as bronchospasm or collapse following the injection of intravenous agents such as thiopentone (thiopental) or althesin which is a mixture of alphadolone (alfadolone) and alphaxalone (alfaxolone) are avoided by choosing local analgesia.

Disadvantages of local analgesia

THE PATIENT'S RESPONSE

Many patients have a fear of injections. Every patient is different, and what one patient considers to be an advantage in a particular technique may be regarded as a disadvantage by another. For example, one may prefer to avoid premedication so that he is not drowsy at the end of the procedure. On the other hand, lack of premedication sometimes results in jumpiness, anxiety, and apprehension, and he may be so frightened before and during the operation that he eventually states that he would never willingly undergo the same again.

AWARENESS

Most patients prefer to be asleep when undergoing surgery. Their being awake during the operation may be distressing because every touch or sensation is sometimes wrongly attributed to lack of pain relief. Consequently the patient loses confidence in his attending medical staff. Any instruction by the attendants in nursing or surgical techniques during the operative period is inadvisable, and can instill fear into the patient.

Certain groups of patients are unsuitable for operative procedures under local analgesia. Lack of co-operation may occur due to spasticity or mental abnormality, or occur in children who frighten easily and whose confidence and subsequent co-operation are difficult to regain. Failure to co-operate is also found in emotionally unstable adults.

ASSOCIATED CONDITIONS

(1) *Bleeding tendencies*
Patients with bleeding tendencies are best excluded, because if the needle used to inject the local analgesic solution inadvertently penetrates a blood vessel, bruising or hematoma formation occurs. Natural causes of bleeding include hemophilia (factor VIII deficiency) and Christmas disease (factor IX deficiency). Therapeutic causes of bleeding are due to treatment with anticoagulants such as warfarin.

(2) *Infection*
Acute inflammation or abscess formation makes the local analgesic solution less effective and there is a risk that infection may be spread through fascial planes with the introduction of the needle. However, nerve blocks performed remote from the operation site, e.g. for the incision and drainage of a paronychia, do not pose this problem.

(3) *Possible overdosage*
Multiple operating sites, and certainly extensive procedures such as suturing of a large laceration in the skin, are generally considered as contra-indications to the use of local analgesia; the large amounts of analgesic solution required carry a risk of overdosage.

(4) *Adverse reactions*
Some patients react adversely to the actual local analgesic solution used. Nerve damage can occur from direct trauma caused by the needle, or by injection of local analgesic solution directly into the nerve itself.

Giving the local analgesic
EQUIPMENT
Most Accident and Emergency departments provide presterilized basic packs containing two paper towels, a gallipot, cotton wool balls, and two pairs of plastic forceps. Additional requirements are sterile disposable 2 ml, 10 ml, or 20 ml syringes and needles, gloves for the surgeon or anesthetist, and an appropriate antiseptic solution, such as chlorhexidine, or a mixture of chlorhexidine and cetrimide.

All anesthetics, whether general or local, should be given in an area of the hospital which contains a tipping chair, trolley (gurney) or table, a sucker, an oxygen source from cylinders or wall supply, an Ambu-bag (p. 224) or some other means of inflating the patient's lungs (p. 222), airways, a sphygmomanometer, an emergency drug box and infusion apparatus, the butterfly type of intravenous needle, Esmarch bandages and Spencer Wells forceps. The presence of adequately trained nursing staff is essential.

Local analgesic drugs

HISTORY

Cocaine was the first agent used for local analgesia, being introduced into medical practice by Karl Koller in 1884. It is extremely toxic and is no longer given by injection; lignocaine (lidocaine) and bupivacaine are considered superior. Lignocaine was synthesized in 1943 by Löfgren and Lundqvist; Ekstam and his colleagues synthesized bupivacaine in 1957.

MODE OF ACTION OF ANALGESIC DRUGS

A local analgesic drug works by penetrating the nerve around which it is injected. It prevents the passage of the nervous impulse or 'action potential' along that nerve, thus producing a 'nerve block'. The speed of onset and ultimate depth of analgesia depend on a number of factors. Firstly, the strength of the solution used is important because the greater the concentration of drug the greater is the degree of penetration or diffusion of that solution into the nerve tissue. Secondly, they depend on the accuracy with which the solution is applied to the nerve in question. The all too familiar expression 'Oh, the local didn't work properly' is a case of a poor workman blaming his tools. All analgesic solutions work properly if they are given correctly, although local infection reduces their efficacy.

Lignocaine and bupivacaine are available as plain or adrenaline containing solutions. Prilocaine is popular in some hospitals, and is often recommended for the Bier's perfusion block (p. 112).

WHY DO SOME ANALGESIC SOLUTIONS CONTAIN ADRENALINE (EPINEPHRINE)?

Adrenaline (epinephrine) is a vasoconstricting drug and a potent stimulator of the sympathetic nervous system, causing marked tachycardia, palpitations, anxiety and sweating (p. 125). These symptoms sometimes occur following the injection of a local analgesic containing adrenaline. However, adrenaline usually in a 1:200 000 concentration, is sometimes added because it prolongs the action of any local analgesic with which it is mixed, and minimizes the risk of toxicity of the analgesic agent by decreasing its rate of absorption into the blood-stream.

At this point it is important to note that the strength of the adrenaline solution in the emergency drug box is 1:1000 (1 mg/ml). The 1:200 000 concentration, as in the preparations labelled 'lignocaine with adrenaline 1:200 000' or 'bupivacaine with adrenaline 1:200 000' is 200 times weaker than that found in the emergency drug box. A 1:1000 solution of adrenaline must never be diluted and added to a plain solution of a local analgesic, lest an error be made in the dilution and an excessive amount of adrenaline injected, with possibly disastrous consequences.

DURATION OF ACTION

A 1% plain lignocaine (lidocaine) solution provides an analgesic block for 1 hour; 1% lignocaine with 1:200 000 adrenaline is effective for 1½–2 hours.

Bupivacaine is four times as potent as lignocaine, has a greater safety margin, and has a duration of block of 5 16 hours. There is nothing to be gained by mixing lignocaine and bupivacaine solutions.

TOXIC EFFECTS

Toxic effects may result from inadvertent intravenous injection, overdosage or rapid absorption. Local analgesic solutions may be absorbed more rapidly from some tissues than others, due to the differences in local blood supply. For example, the rate of absorption from an intercostal injection is greater than that from subcutaneous infiltration of the abdominal wall.

Local analgesic techniques

The nurse plays an important part in guaranteeing the success of various operative procedures performed under local analgesia, and should therefore be familiar with their practical application. The procedures carried out in the Accident and Emergency department include:

(1) cleaning of abrasions
(2) suturing of lacerations and occasionally tendons (p. 18)
(3) reduction of fractures such as Colles', Smith's, mid-shaft radius and ulna, and digits (p. 64)
(4) removal of fingernails or toenails (p. 101)
(5) the siting of intravenous cannulae before the patient is admitted to the wards

(6)   incision and drainage of abscesses, bearing in mind the dangers
      mentioned on page 107.

MANAGEMENT OF THE PATIENT
A sympathetic and unhurried approach often helps to relax or reassure
an apprehensive patient. An air of calm efficiency more than
compensates for the absence of some form of premedication.
Persuading an unwilling patient to accept local analgesia is often
associated with only partial analgesia, increasing discomfort, fear and
distrust. It is helpful to talk to him, explaining what will be done, and
reassure him that it will not hurt. Having to keep still for a long time is
often difficult, especially with old people who may suffer from cramp
or arthritis. If the environment is cool or draughty, the patient must be
kept well covered, but care is taken to avoid smothering him with sterile
towels or drapes placed around the face. Separate coverings are also
necessary to maintain decency and avoid embarrassment. It is wise to
avoid joking or arguing between nursing and medical staff, and talking
about other patients or operations. The nurse should have the suction
apparatus available, and watch for retching or vomiting during the
procedure.

Local analgesia may be classified as follows:

   (a)   surface or topical analgesia
   (b)   infiltration
   (c)   nerve blocks
   (d)   intravenous perfusion

   Surface or topical analgesia is useful for work on the cornea, on
mucous membranes and abrasions, but not on unbroken skin which
prevents the penetration, and therefore the action, of local analgesics.
Corneal foreign bodies can be removed using 1% amethocaine
(tetracaine).

Skin abrasions
Grazes are often contaminated with dirt, and need to be washed and
cleaned; 5% lignocaine gel smeared over the graze allows the area to be
easily brushed with an aqueous solution of cetrimide or chlorhexidine.

Lacerations
The skin surrounding the wound can be anesthetized by the subcutaneous infiltration of local analgesic solution (Figure 13.1). Most
operators use a 25 G 16 mm long needle to raise the initial skin bleb, and
follow through this anesthetized patch of skin with a larger bore 23 G

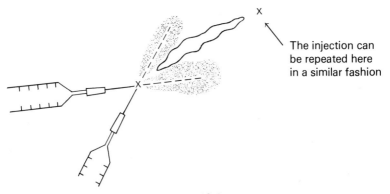

The injection can be repeated here in a similar fashion

Figure 13.1

needle. The injection of local analgesic solution under the edge of the wound is less painful for the patient but is carried out through a potentially contaminated area.

It is essential, especially when injecting local analgesics prior to suturing facial lacerations, to ensure that the needle is firmly attached to the syringe, otherwise the sudden gush of analgesic solution over patient and operator tends to alarm both.

Although the maximum dose of analgesic solution is seldom reached during the suturing of most wounds, the temptation to exceed it must be resisted, and multiple or major lacerations should be dealt with under a general anaesthetic.

DANGERS OF LOCAL ANALGESIC WITH ADRENALINE SOLUTIONS

Adrenaline-containing solutions help to reduce the risk of toxicity but they should never be used when treating end-organs, such as the penis, fingers and toes. The blood supply to these end-organs is through an end-artery, which is the terminal branch of the arterial supply to the organ which has no collateral circulation. Consequently any vaso-constriction caused in these structures may produce local ischemia, tissue anoxia and tissue death (gangrene).

REMOVAL OF TOURNIQUETS

After every procedure, the utmost vigilance is necessary to confirm that no rubber band or other type of tourniquet has been left in position. If these are left on until the dressings are applied, they may be forgotten, with disastrous results. The patient will be unaware of the presence of the tourniquet because he will have no pain until the local analgesic wears off a few hours later. By the time the mistake is discovered, irreversible anoxic changes may have occurred.

BIER'S BLOCK (INTRAVENOUS REGIONAL ANALGESIA)
History
August Bier in 1908 intravenously injected a dilute solution of procaine *between* two tourniquets placed above and below the elbow of a girl suffering from severe tuberculosis of the elbow. Bier's technique was occasionally associated with the toxic effects of procaine, but nowadays this intravenous perfusion technique is performed by injecting lignocaine, bupivacaine, or prilocaine distally to a special pneumatic double tourniquet, or two sphygmomanometer cuffs acting as tourniquets, inflated above the level of the patient's systolic blood pressure.

Indications
With the Bier technique good analgesia and muscle relaxation can be obtained to allow the reduction of forearm bone fractures, and the suturing of tendons and wounds.

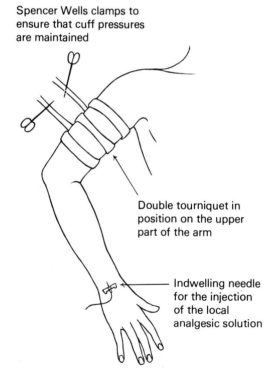

Spencer Wells clamps to
ensure that cuff pressures
are maintained

Double tourniquet in
position on the upper
part of the arm

Indwelling needle
for the injection
of the local
analgesic solution

Figure 13.2

Details of the technique

The patient's weight, blood pressure and pulse rate are recorded. A 23 G butterfly needle is inserted into a vein on the dorsum of the injured hand, and either a special double tourniquet or two ordinary sphygmomanometer cuffs are placed around the upper arm. The limb is exsanguinated by wrapping a rubber Esmarch bandage around the arm, starting at the finger tips and working proximally as far as the tourniquet. A painful Colles' fracture makes the effective application of the Esmarch bandage almost impossible but elevation for a short time is usually a satisfactory alternative. The proximal tourniquet is next inflated to at least 50 mmHg above the systolic blood pressure and the calculated dose of local analgesic solution is injected through the indwelling needle. As this is done, the skin around the needle site becomes quite blotchy. The onset of analgesia occurs within 5–10 minutes. Then the distal tourniquet or cuff is inflated to the same pressure as the upper one (Figure 13.2), which is then deflated, leaving the remaining tight cuff over the insensitive upper arm.

It is important to note the time when the tourniquet is applied, and to watch the cuff or tourniquet pressures continuously during the procedure in case they drop significantly. It is also essential to observe the patient carefully after release of the tourniquet at the end of the procedure because if side-effects occur they demand urgent treatment (p. 116). As a precaution, the author always inserts a second butterfly needle in the uninjured hand in case resuscitative drugs are required. Some patients receiving lignocaine show signs of the systemic effects (p. 115) of the drug, whereas this is much less likely to occur with bupivacaine.

BRACHIAL PLEXUS BLOCK

The brachial plexus, from which arise the median, radial and ulnar nerves supplying the arm, can be approached by either the supraclavicular or the axillary route.

Supraclavicular approach

The major disadvantage of this method is that the pleura or lung can be accidentally punctured during the injection of local analgesic solution causing a pneumothorax. Pleural puncture is painful and may make the patient cough. Anyone who becomes breathless after a supraclavicular brachial plexus block should be considered to have a pneumothorax, which can usually but not always be confirmed by a chest X-ray. Even if the X-ray is normal the patient should be admitted to hospital overnight as a precautionary measure, and a repeat chest X-ray taken before his discharge, lest a slowly developing pneumothorax be missed. A small pneumothorax requires no special treatment because the air is slowly reabsorbed. A large pneumothorax or a tension pneumothorax decrease the available effective lung volume, and may cause severe respiratory embarrassment, shift the mediastinum, reduce the cardiac output, and need treatment with an underwater-seal chest drain (p. 267).

Axillary approach to the brachial plexus
The great advantage of the axillary approach to the brachial plexus is the absence of any risk of pleural damage. Local analgesic solution can be injected into the fascial sheath surrounding the axillary artery and branches of the brachial plexus through a 23 G butterfly intermittent infusion set, the rubber seal having been removed from the end (Figure 13.3). Introduction of the local analgesic solution in this way, remote from the needle itself, ensures that the needle does not move either during the injection of the analgesic solution or during the changing of syringes which is necessary because up to 30 ml of 0.5% plain bupivacaine may be required. It also allows aspiration to check that the needle tip does not lie within a vessel. If it does, there will be free flow of bright red arterial, or darker venous, blood along the plastic tubing.

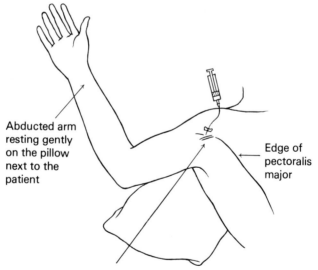

Abducted arm resting gently on the pillow next to the patient

Edge of pectoralis major

Axillary artery palpated and the butterfly needle inserted above, and as close to, the artery as possible

Figure 13.3

No local analgesic works instantly. 20–30 minutes often elapse before the block works adequately, after which a variety of operations on the hand, forearm, and distal part of the upper arm are possible. At all times the patient's comments are considered correct; if he says he is in pain, he must be believed. Sometimes, 5–15 mg diazepam, an excellent tranquillizing drug, is given by slow intravenous injection into a large vein, usually in the antecubital fossa, because it allows the patient to relax, and confers some degree of anterograde amnesia, which means that the patient's memory is hazy from the time of the injection onwards.

AFTER CARE
The patient is warned, before he leaves the hospital, that the pain might return as the effect of the local analgesic wears off. He is also told that after a brachial plexus block, for example, the arm could be insensitive to pain or heat for up to 16 hours if bupivacaine has been used. Holding a hot water bottle against a forearm plaster during this time, to expedite the drying of the plaster of Paris, has resulted in burns being caused because the patient is unaware that the hot water bottle is too hot. Most painful conditions at home usually respond to treatment with mild analgesic preparations such as 1 G paracetamol (acetaminophen), 600 mg soluble aspirin, 60 mg dihydrocodeine, 250 mg diflunisal, or a mixture of 325 mg paracetamol and 32.5 mg dextropropoxyphene. Immobilization or elevation, if this is appropriate, often alleviates pain.

Complications associated with local analgesia
Although local analgesia is usually safer than general anesthesia, complications do occur; some are serious and require immediate treatment. Complications due to toxic reactions to the analgesic solution can be systemic or local in nature.

SYSTEMIC OR GENERAL COMPLICATIONS
The level of local analgesic drug in the bloodstream determines whether a toxic reaction occurs. Accidental intravascular injection, which gives a high blood level, an actual overdosage, or rapid absorption may be associated with the patient complaining of lightheadedness, tingling around the lips and tongue, a metallic taste in the mouth, or visual disturbances such as the sensation that objects in the room are beginning to move. He may show signs ranging from pallor and muscular twitching to unconsciousness, convulsions, respiratory depression or respiratory arrest. Respiratory depression can arise not only from the toxic effect of the analgesic solution on the pons and

medulla in the midbrain but also by excessive dosage of tranquillizing or analgesic drugs used concurrently, such as diazepam or morphine. Ultimately cardiovascular depression occurs, with hypotension, bradycardia, and finally cardiac arrest and death.

Treatment of the complications
Treatment is directed towards abolishing hypoxia, stopping convulsions and reversing the circulatory depression, which is itself aggravated by hypoxia.

The patient with severe respiratory depression invariably requires artificial ventilation with oxygen, using a Brook airway, Ambu-bag and a face mask (p. 224), or the Magill circuit (p. 202 and 203) on an anesthetic machine. Intubation of the trachea may be necessary later.

Intravenous diazepam 10–20 mg or thiopentone (thiopental) 50–150 mg are excellent anticonvulsant drugs. Repeated doses can be given should convulsions recur. Suxamethonium (succinylcholine p. 219) is a short-acting muscle relaxant without any hypnotic properties; 50–100 mg given intravenously stops the muscle contractions which occur during the convulsions. The resulting respiratory paralysis requires immediate and sustained intermittent positive pressure ventilation. Suxamethonium should not be given to a conscious patient, and should be preceded by an anticonvulsant (p. 258).

Hypotension may respond to elevating the patient's legs, adopting a head-down tilt with the table, or by injecting a suitable vasopressor, such as 5–15 mg ephedrine or 5–10 mg methoxamine intravenously. Atropine 0.5–1 mg should be given intravenously if bradycardia is present. If cardiac arrest is suspected, with absent pulse, unconsciousness, absent respiration and dilated pupils, external cardiac massage should be started immediately (p. 261).

LOCAL COMPLICATIONS
These include:

(1) Tissue reactions to metallic ions in the solution, resulting in edema formation.
(2) Infection. This is usually the result of inadequate or absent antiseptic precautions.
(3) Hematoma formation (p. 36).
(4) Ischemia, necrosis and gangrene following the use of adrenaline containing solutions in organs supplied by end-arteries.
(5) Failure to check the contents of the ampule of the drugs used.
(6) Needle breakage during an injection; they should usually be recovered.

RESUMÉ OF THE TREATMENT OF COMPLICATIONS
(a) *Without cardiac arrest:*
Control the airway
Give oxygen
Assist ventilation if necessary
Place the patient in the coma position (p. 180)
Give anticonvulsant
Record the ECG (EKG)
Set up an intravenous infusion if dysrhythmias are present.

(b) *When cardiac arrest has occurred:*
Control the airway
Give oxygen
Assist ventilation
Start external cardiac massage
Record the ECG (EKG)
Set up the intravenous infusion, to give 8.4% sodium bicarbonate, cardiac drugs, or anticonvulsants.

14

Blood pressure regulation

F. WILSON

At some time or other during her stay in the Accident and Emergency department the nurse will assist in maintaining or restoring a patient's blood pressure. Hypotension can be caused by many different conditions ranging from the effects of severe trauma to those of coronary occlusion. In order to appreciate the principles behind the various types of treatment she should be familiar with the factors which maintain normal blood pressure, the way the body compensates in response to injury or disease and the methods by which the blood pressure can be restored.

The heart

The heart consists of four chambers, namely the left atrium and left ventricle, together constituting the left side of the heart, and the right atrium and right ventricle which form the right side of the heart. The thin walled atria are best regarded as acting principally as receiving chambers, the left receiving oxygenated blood from the lungs via the pulmonary veins and the right receiving the de-oxygenated blood from the tissues through the superior and inferior venae cavae (SVC and IVC). The latter two large veins are often referred to as the *great veins* and the pressure in them is referred to as the central venous pressure (CVP). This pressure is measured by means of a CVP line (p. 137 – Figure 15.2), which consists of a catheter introduced into one of the smaller veins and guided along until it enters the SVC. CVP line readings are valuable when infusing intravenous fluids and indicate to the doctor the volume he should infuse.

At this stage it must be understood that although it is customary to measure the central venous pressure (CVP) in the SVC rather than the IVC, any factor which influences the SVC pressure equally influences that in the IVC; therefore any future reference to the SVC regarding pressure changes and venous return refers equally to those in the IVC.

THE PRE-LOAD

When the heart relaxes, that is, when it is in diastole the blood already waiting in the venae cavae flows into the receiving chamber, namely the right atrium. Then, still in diastole, the blood flows from the atrium to the thicker walled pumping chamber or ventricle through the atrio-ventricular valve until diastole ends.

At the end of diastole, because the quantity of blood awaiting expulsion is loaded up in the right ventricular cavity it is known as the pre-load. Normally an equal pre-load, delivered by the pulmonary veins from the lungs (p. 268), exists also on the left side of the heart.

The pre-load depends on the return of blood, on the right side, by the venae cavae. If there is insufficient venous return to the heart then the pre-load is reduced, a diminished output of blood results and the blood pressure falls. On the other hand excessive transfusion increases venous return too much causing an overlarge pre-load which distends the ventricular wall to such an extent that it is unable to function properly and is incapable of emptying itself completely. Eventually the extra effort involved in trying to empty too full a ventricle causes fatigue of the cardiac muscle which then fails in its objective, so the patient develops cardiac failure with a rising pressure in the large veins entering the heart. Failure of the right side of the heart for any reason causes peripheral edema and hepatic congestion but tends to develop more slowly and insidiously than left-sided heart failure which usually becomes clinically obvious as pulmonary edema (see below p. 120).

Our knowledge of pre-loads combined with the help of a CVP line can be very useful to the doctor, particularly when fluid replacement is needed in a patient whose cardiac function is under suspicion (p. 138).

VENTRICULAR SYSTOLE

This can be explained by considering what happens to the contents of the right ventricle. At the start of systole the atrioventricular valve closes, preventing blood passing back into the right atrium. Simultaneously the valve between the right ventricle and the pulmonary artery opens allowing the blood to eject into the pulmonary artery and enter the lungs. Leaving the lungs via the pulmonary veins the oxygenated blood enters the left atrium, passes into the left ventricle and is forced by left ventricular systole into the aorta which directs the oxygenated blood into the tissues (Figure 14.1). It can be seen, therefore, that the heart really consists of two pumps side by side which must function in complete co-operation with each other because the blood they pump is common to both. This unique arrangement sometimes breaks down in disease and any disturbance in function of one side of the system usually affects the other. If, for example, the left side of the heart fails to function adequately it is unable to effectively

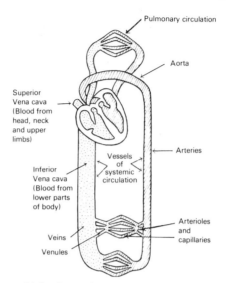

Figure 14.1 Systemic and pulmonary circulations

discharge its blood from the pulmonary veins, which become congested as do the smaller veins in the lungs which lead into them. Consequently, some of the contents of the congested capillaries escape through their walls and produce the pink frothy sputum of 'pulmonary edema'. The lung congestion prevents complete emptying of the right side of the heart and eventually right ventricular failure supervenes, with a rising systemic venous pressure and peripheral edema. In such circumstances the treatment is designed to help the failing heart recover its efficiency, the specific therapy depending on the causative factors. Examples of disturbances in the balance of the two sides of the cardiovascular system and their treatment in the Accident and Emergency department are discussed later (p. 259).

The blood pressure (BP)

At the same time as the pre-load exists in the right ventricle a similar quantity of blood resides in the left ventricle. During ventricular contraction this left ventricular blood enters the aorta: the sudden surge of blood causes the pressure to rise in the aorta and its divisions. The highest reading obtainable at this stage is known as the systolic blood pressure, and is measured on the sphygmomanometer at the instant the nurse hears the sounds start to come through her stethoscope which is placed over the brachial artery at the front of the elbow.

At the end of systole the aortic valve between the left ventricle and the aorta closes to prevent blood flowing back into the heart when the ventricle starts to relax (diastole). Although during diastole no blood is pumped into the arteries their elastic walls squeeze some of their contained blood further into the vascular tree towards the tissues. As more and more blood flows into the tissues the blood pressure in the arteries starts to fall and does so until the next surge of blood enters from the next heart beat. There is, therefore, a moment of time at which the pressure in the arteries is at its lowest. The pressure at this instant is known as the diastolic pressure which is therefore the pressure in the arteries at the end of diastole. This is recorded when the beats heard through the stethoscope just begin to fade (become muffled) or disappear, or both. Obviously the value obtained for the diastolic pressure when measured as the beats begin to fade is higher than that measured as the sounds disappear. Therefore the nurse should always state on the patient's chart which criterion she adopts when recording the diastolic blood pressure.

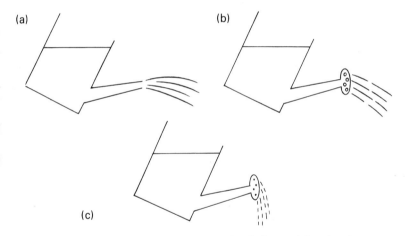

Figure 14.2 Flow from watering cans simulating peripheral resistance

PERIPHERAL RESISTANCE
The meaning and significance of peripheral resistance may be illustrated by the use of three watering cans (Figure 14.2a–c).

(a) Can A has no rose and when tilted it empties in 1 second.
(b) If can B, which has a rose, is tilted for 1 second some of the water escapes but some is left behind because the dozens of small tubes in the substance of the rose resist the passage of the water through them. The can may be regarded as the aorta, the spout as a large artery, and the little tubes whose mouths appear as holes in the rose may be looked

upon as the arterioles. Therefore, small tubes resist the flow of fluid through them much more than wider tubes, i.e. they have a greater resistance. Another example of the resistance of a narrow tube is demonstrated if the nurse sees how quickly she can empty a 20 ml syringe through a wide bore needle, and compare it with the emptying time through a small bore. It is obvious that the resistance to flow through the small bore needle is much the greater of the two. This is why the arterioles, combined with the fact that they are situated peripherally, produce or constitute what is known as the peripheral resistance.

(c)   The rose of can C has smaller holes than that of can B, and if both are tilted equally the water emerges from B as a spray but just manages to dribble out from can C. Therefore, if the peripheral resistance of the arterioles is increased too much, that is if arteriolar constriction is too profound, they may not deliver sufficient blood to the tissues. Consequently, the flow of blood through them, i.e. the perfusion, may be insufficient to provide the cells with adequate oxygen, thus causing tissue damage or death.

From the above discussion and experiments it is obvious that the arteries contain blood at the end of diastole, and there must be a reason why they do not empty completely. This can be explained, that as the arteries divide into smaller and smaller vessels eventually becoming arterioles, their lumina become so narrow that the blood can only pass through them slowly. In other words, although the arterioles permit blood to flow through them, they constitute a resistance to the blood flowing from the larger arteries into the tissues.

Low peripheral resistance
If the arterioles dilate due to a drug or disease, the blood from the arteries escapes too fast into the tissues, which fill like a sponge. As a result the diastolic pressure drops, and the heart may not have sufficient time, power or supply of blood entering it to refill the arteries. Consequently, the systolic pressure also falls and the patient may faint due to lack of a blood supply to the brain. A situation has therefore arisen where there is insufficient blood in the vascular system to maintain an adequate pressure, despite the fact that no blood has been lost to the outside of the body. This discrepancy can be corrected by blood transfusion or by causing the arterioles to contract, so that just like squeezing a sponge their contents are restored to the general circulation.

The result, in health, is that the elastic and muscle tissue in the arteries and the arterioles continue to squeeze their contained blood during diastole and keep a continuous and adequate flow of blood into the tissues throughout the cardiac cycle.

High peripheral resistance

Because the peripheral resistance constitutes a load against which the heart must pump its blood, it is sometimes referred to as the 'after-load'. If the left ventricle is at the point of failure and the after-load is increased by constriction of the arterioles with an alpha-receptor (p. 125) stimulating agent, the extra work may be too much so that the ventricle fails completely. Furthermore, excessive arteriolar constriction can 'shut down' the arterioles, thus cutting off the blood supply to the tissues.

It can be seen, therefore. that arteriolar constriction is a double-edged weapon; it helps to produce and maintain a blood pressure sufficient to ensure adequate tissue perfusion but, if over-zealous, the constriction becomes too much and threatens the blood supply to the tissues.

SELECTIVE SHUTDOWN OF ARTERIOLES

The body uses its arterioles to ensure an adequate supply of blood to its vital organs very effectively especially when bleeding occurs. Loss of blood from say a traffic accident reduces the blood volume which, unless compensatory mechanisms come into play, causes a fall in blood pressure. The response of the body is to maintain the blood supply to vital organs such as the brain and heart, which it ensures by leaving their arterioles open. On the other hand, it almost completely closes the arterioles supplying the skin and gut whose contained blood is squeezed into the circulation, thereby maintaining the blood pressure but at the cost of a diminished blood supply to themselves. This explains why the skin of a patient who has bled, or is bleeding, is pale and cold. If eventually his compensatory mechanisms begin to fail and his blood pressure falls, he is said to have 'cold hypotension'. If such a person is warmed too quickly, his skin vessels dilate and admit blood so that less is available for his vital tissues, and his condition will worsen. This is why a shocked person should be prevented from getting cold but should not be overheated.

BLOOD PRESSURE (BP) AND CARDIAC OUTPUT

The heart can only pump into the aorta blood which has previously been returned to it by the great veins. Therefore, the cardiac output depends on and is in fact equal to the venous return, and because maintenance of the blood pressure depends on the arteries having adequate blood inside them it is obvious that blood pressure must, to some extent, depend on the cardiac output.

However, it has already been stated that the peripheral resistance influences the blood pressure and so it is obvious that blood pressure depends on the cardiac output and the peripheral resistance. Actually blood pressure is defined as being equal to the product of the cardiac output and the peripheral resistance, that is

blood pressure = cardiac output × peripheral resistance.

Effect of cardiac output on the BP
The volume of blood ejected by each ventricle per minute depends on how much blood it squirts out per beat (about 80 ml) and the number of beats it performs per minute (about 70).

∴ $\dfrac{\text{Cardiac output}}{\text{in ml per minute}} = \dfrac{\text{volume discharged}}{\text{per beat in ml}}$ × number of beats per minute

∴ In the above example:

the cardiac output = (80 × 70) ml/min
= 5600 ml/min
= 5.6 l/min

If the cardiac output falls because there is insufficient blood in the cardiovascular system, as occurs following severe hemorrhage, then the blood pressure would fall were it not for the arterioles increasing the peripheral resistance.

Therefore, following hemorrhage the BP remains within normal limits if the cardiac output falls, provided that the peripheral resistance increases. Similarly, if the peripheral resistance falls, the blood pressure can be maintained by increasing the cardiac output; the heart beats faster and pushes the circulating blood quicker than usual round the body, i.e. there is a reduced circulatory time.

Therefore, if the left ventricle pumps out 80 ml/beat at a rate of 90 beats/min,

the cardiac output = (80 × 90) ml/min
= 7200 ml/min
= 7.2 l/min.

However, there is a limit to the rate at which the heart can beat and push the blood to and through the tissues; if the blood volume falls too much there is a diminished venous return to the heart. Since the ventricles cannot pump out what they do not receive, the cardiac output falls and if the peripheral resistance cannot increase sufficiently to compensate for the reduced blood volume, the BP falls further and may become unrecordable. Eventually there is insufficient blood in the circulation to maintain adequate tissue perfusion and the patient dies.

RESPONSE OF THE BODY TO BLOOD LOSS
Whenever blood is lost, the response of the body is to try to maintain

the blood pressure by increasing both the peripheral resistance and the cardiac output. The skin becomes pale and the heart rate increases. Such a response depends on the activity of the sympathetic nervous system whose main centres of action are near to each other in the medulla of the brain. From these centres, respectively called the cardiac accelerator centre and the vasomotor-centre, sympathetic nerve fibres pass to the heart and the blood vessels. Usually they help to maintain the heart rate and the calibre of the arteries and arterioles within normal limits so that the blood pressure remains stable. However, if blood is lost there is increased activity in the nerves leaving the cardiac accelerator centre so that the heart rate rises, and also in the sympathetic fibres leaving the vasomotor centre which increase the peripheral resistance. The adrenal medulla is also stimulated.

Such a response is due to the effect of the chemical transmitters adrenaline (epinephrine) and noradrenaline (norepinephrine). Following blood loss the blood pressure tends to fall and this change is detected by sensitive nerve endings (pressure or baroreceptors) in the carotid arteries. As a result the information is conveyed to the cardiac accelerator and vasomotor centres and from them the message, in the form of nerve impulses, is passed down to the ends of those sympathetic fibres in intimate contact with the cells of the heart and blood vessels.

On arrival at the nerve endings the impulses liberate chemical substances such as noradrenaline and adrenaline which transmit the message by chemical attachment to special receptors on the cardiac and arteriolar muscle cells which respond by making the muscle fibres contract. The noradrenaline and adrenaline are referred to as chemical transmitters, and because when injected they produce a response which *mimics* those produced by stimulating the sympathetic nerves they are said to have a sympatho*mimetic* action. Because these transmitters have an $[-NH_2]$ group, known as the amine group, in their chemical structure they are also known as the sympathomimetic amines.

Alpha (α) and beta (β)-receptors
Above it was stated that the sympathomimetic amines act on special receptors. These receptors on the cells in the heart are known as beta one-receptors (β_1) and those in the arterioles as alpha (α)-receptors. Stimulation of β_1-receptors on the heart causes the heart to beat faster and stronger and so helps to increase cardiac output. Stimulation of alpha-receptors causes the arterioles to contract and the peripheral resistance to increase and so help to maintain the blood pressure.

Drugs which stimulate α-receptors are known as α-adrenoreceptor agonists and those that stimulate β-receptors are called β-adreno-receptor agonists.

The response of these receptors is obvious whenever the body is prepared for 'fight or flight'. If a person is afraid or involved in fighting the sympathetic nervous system immediately responds by increasing the heart rate and reducing the blood supply to the skin so that pallor is apparent. Other effects of sympathetic overactivity take place such as the breathing becomes more rapid, sweating occurs and the bronchi and pupils dilate. The receptors in the bronchi which produce bronchial dilatation are known as beta two (β_2)-receptors.

There are drugs which principally stimulate all three, that is α, β_1 and β_2-receptors and others that stimulate only β_1 and β_2 or just β_1 or β_2 or α-receptors.

Before discussing the use of sympathomimetic drugs it is necessary to mention the relationship between the sympathetic nervous system and the parasympathetic nervous system. Basically, whatever one does the other does the opposite, for example:

Organ	Effect of sympathetic action	Effect of parasympathetic action
Heart	Heart rate up	Heart rate down
Eye	Pupil dilates	Pupil contracts
Bronchi	Dilate	Constrict

There is, therefore, a balance between the two which moderates the actions of the various organs, so that a happy medium is reached which is suitable for normal body activity. For example, besides the sympathetic nerve supply to the heart, stimulation of which increases the heart rate, there is also a parasympathetic nerve supply (the vagus nerves) whose action is to slow it down. The heart rate at any particular moment depends on which type of nerve action is predominant. In health the vagus usually predominates.

Several varieties of drugs are available which can increase or decrease the actions of the sympathetic and parasympathetic nervous systems. They are divided into four main groups.

(1) Sympathomimetic drugs increase sympathetic activity: they include the α and β-receptor agonists (p. 128).
(2) Sympatholytic drugs decrease sympathetic activity: they include the blockers (p. 127).
(3) Parasympathomimetic drugs increase parasympathetic activity.
(4) Parasympatholytic drugs decrease parasympathetic activity.

When it is desirable to raise the heart rate, a sympathomimetic drug may be used to increase the sympathetic effect on the heart, thus overpowering the influence of the vagus nerves. Alternatively, a parasympatholytic drug may be selected to reduce the influence of the vagus nerves thereby causing less slowing of the heart, which is another way of saying that it allows the heart to beat faster, because the sympathetic action is then unopposed. Those of us who have had a tooth extracted under local analgesia, such as lignocaine with adrenaline (lidocaine with epinephrine) or a general anesthetic with an atropine-containing premedication will recall the increased heart rate which ensued, usually accompanied by palpitations. Adrenaline is a sympathomimetic type of drug whereas atropine has a parasympatholytic effect – yet their action on the heart rate is similar. However, both these drugs, like others with similar actions, have side-effects which maybe unpleasant, unwanted and even dangerous. Therefore, the doctor has to decide which type of drug produces the specific action he requires with minimal side-effects. If he wants to increase the heart rate he usually uses atropine. Although this gives the patient a dry mouth it is less unpleasant than the excitement or jitters produced by most of the sympathomimetic group of drugs.

THE USE OF BLOCKERS

Noradrenaline is the chemical transmitter which acts at most sympathetic nerve endings. However, at most of the parasympathetic nerve endings a different chemical transmitter is involved known as acetylcholine which is also involved in and necessary for initiating and maintaining the contractions of the voluntary muscles.

All of these transmitters act on the receptors of specific tissues; for example, stimulation of β_1-receptors increases the heart rate and β_2-stimulation dilates the bronchi whereas α-stimulation increases the peripheral resistance (p. 121). These receptors are constantly being stimulated in normal life and therefore if they can be blocked, so that the transmitter cannot occupy them, then the tissue on which they act will no longer be under their influence. Drugs are available which do this – they block the receptors and are therefore called adrenoreceptor blocking agents or just 'blockers'. A β-adrenoreceptor blocking agent such as propranolol blocks the effects of both β_1 and β_2-stimulation, so that the chemical transmitters which stimulate the heart rate and dilate the bronchi are rendered less effective and the result is that the heart slows and the bronchi constrict. Fortunately the effect of propranolol on the bronchi is usually negligible but care is necessary in asthma, chronic bronchitis and emphysema. Oxprenolol is said to have a more selective blocking action than propranolol on β_1-receptors and consequently causes less bronchial constriction.

The α-adrenoreceptor blocking agents are used infrequently as they cause the arterioles to dilate and the peripheral resistance and the blood pressure to fall. The α-blocker phentolamine is sometimes used when hypertension is caused by too much adrenaline and noradrenaline being produced, such as occurs in the presence of a tumour of the adrenal glands, known as a phaeochromocytoma. On occasions, it is used in severe shock, to reduce vasoconstriction and increase tissue perfusion when the circulatory blood volume has been replaced, but it is unlikely to be used in the Accident and Emergency department.

The Accident and Emergency nurse will often meet patients who are taking β_1-blockers. They are usually prescribed for angina or hypertensive heart disease. Slowing the heart reduces its work and may be effective in reducing the incidence or severity of the angina. Therefore, the likelihood of heart disease should be considered in anyone on β-blockers who requires anesthesia. Special precautions may have to be taken and indeed local analgesia (p. 104) may often be safer.

The β-blockers are sometimes given in emergency situations where restoration of the heart rate towards normal levels may become urgent, e.g. in a life-threatening tachycardia. Such drugs are used in cardiac conditions, and must not be used to try to reduce the tachycardia due to blood loss, where the proper treatment is to restore the blood volume.

A pure β_2-blocker has not been developed, as there is no clinical use for such a drug; but some β_2-blocking action does occasionally occur as a result of side-effects in the use of drugs with a mainly β_1-blocking action (see above). On the contrary, drugs such as salbutamol, which stimulate the β_2-receptors in the bronchi, are frequently used for their bronchodilator effects in asthma and are usually given by means of a metered aerosol inhaler. Isoprenaline (isoproterenol) is another β_2-stimulant useful in asthma, but as a side-effect also markedly stimulates the β_1-receptors so that the heart rate increases. Some asthmatic patients have overdosed themselves with isoproterenol from inhalers while trying to relieve their symptoms, resulting in the β_1-receptors being overstimulated and leading to death from heart failure. The β effects on the heart are in fact so powerful that the drug is sometimes used intravenously in shock, in an attempt to increase the cardiac output.

Because of the complexity of action of the drugs acting on the sympathetic and parasympathetic nervous systems the nurse may initially prefer to restrict her knowledge to the following:

Combined β_1 and β_2-blockers – propranolol – reduces tachycardia. May reduce angina by allowing heart to function more effectively.

Specific β_1-blockers – oxprenolol – less bronchoconstricting than propranolol.

Specific α-blocker – phentolamine – lowers peripheral resistance.

β_1 and β_2-stimulators – isoprenaline – increases force of contraction and heart rate and therefore may raise the blood pressure.

β_2-stimulators   – salbutamol – dilates bronchi.

Parasympatholytic   – atropine – increases heart rate. May raise blood pressure by increasing cardiac output.

15

Blood volume maintenance and restoration

F. WILSON

Blood volume

The normal blood volume is 80 ml/kg (40*ml/lb) body weight. A child weighing 20 kg (44 lb) has a blood volume of about 1600 ml (1.6 l) whereas the adult weighing 70 kg (150 lb) has a blood volume of approximately 5.6 l. Immediately it is obvious that a loss of 0.5 l of blood in such a child deprives him of one-third of his blood volume and is therefore more serious than the same loss in an adult which amounts to only one-eleventh of his blood volume. Similarly, it is apparent that transfusion of 0.5 l of blood to a child has a much greater chance of overloading his circulation than it has in the adult patient.

Constituents of blood

PLASMA

Plasma is blood without its corpuscles. It contains proteins, which are necessary to prevent its fluid component from seeping completely into the tissues (p. 131), and crystalloids such as sodium, potassium and chloride and many other substances needed for the healthy functioning of the body.

Plasma also carries a small amount of dissolved oxygen.

RED BLOOD CELLS (RBCs)

The function of the RBC is to carry oxygen and carbon dioxide between the lungs and other tissues.

The function of plasma proteins

When blood leaves the arterioles it passes into the capillaries whose walls are deficient in that they allow some of the constituents of plasma

---

*These figures are quoted for easy remembering – they are approximate because 1 kg = 2.2 lb.

to pass into the tissues. However, these 'deficiencies' or holes are only large enough to allow fluid and crystalloids to escape, they are too small to allow the larger protein particles and RBCs to pass out of the capillaries. This interchange of fluids and nutrients is produced by the differences of pressure between the inside and outside of the capillary. Plasma proteins have an osmotic effect which means that they have the ability to suck fluids towards them.

	Hydrostatic pressure (mmHg)	Interstitial fluid pressure (mmHg)	Osmotic pressure of protein (suction pressure) (mmHg)	Result
Start of capillary	36	1	25	35 − 25 = 10 mmHg ∴ fluid passes out of capillary.
Middle of capillary	26	1	25	25 − 25 = 0 mmHg ∴ fluid passes neither in nor out of capillary.
End of capillary	12	1	25	11 − 25 = − 14 mmHg ∴ fluid is sucked back into capillary.

Figure 15.1

Figure 15.1 shows that the pressure exerted by the 'fluid or water' component of the plasma (the hydrostatic pressure) at the junction of an arteriole and the capillary, is 36 mmHg. Due to friction between the cells and plasma and the capillary wall the pressure at the end of the capillary is only 12 mmHg. These hydrostatic pressures try to push the capillary contents through the 'holes' in the capillary lining.

However, outside the capillaries, there is also interstitial fluid in the tissues which exerts a pressure which tries to push fluid from the tissues into the capillaries, but the interstitial pressure has a value of only 1 mmHg. Therefore, at the beginning of the capillary the pressure inside the capillary (the intracapillary pressure) of 36 mmHg is greater than the tissue pressure of 1 mmHg by 36 − 1 mmHg = 35 mmHg, so fluid is pushed into the tissue spaces.

At the distal end of the capillary the hydrostatic pressure is only 12 mmHg, but this is still 11 mmHg greater than the interstitial pressure. If the hydrostatic pressures were the only factors involved in transference of fluid between capillaries and tissues the end result would be that the capillaries would empty and the interstitial tissues would start to and continue to swell. In other words, the capillaries would empty their fluid content into the tissues, none of it would re-enter the capillaries and no fluid constituent of the plasma would return to the heart. That such an event does not happen is due to the suction power (osmotic pressure effect) of the plasma proteins. These proteins exert an osmotic pressure of 25 mmHg which sucks fluid towards them, and so opposes the movement of the fluid from capillaries to tissues. There is a constant battle between the hydrostatic pressure forcing fluid out of the capillaries, and the osmotic pressure of the plasma proteins trying to draw it back. At the start of the capillary (the proximal end) the hydrostatic pressure wins.

In the middle of the capillary there is a stalemate where hydrostatic and osmotic pressures are equal, so little transference of fluid takes place. At the distal end of the capillary the osmotic power of the proteins is greater than the hydrostatic pressure, so fluid is attracted back into the capillary. Therefore, the blood is reconstituted at the distal end of the capillary from which it is returned to the heart.

Membrane permeability

When membranes allow water and crystalloids such as sodium, potassium and chloride to pass through their walls, yet prevent protein particles from doing so, they are regarded as being semi-permeable. Hence, the capillary walls allow the intimate exchange of fluids, crystalloids and dissolved oxygen and carbon dioxide to take place between their enclosed blood and the tissue cells.

If any of the relationships between the pressures in the capillaries and the tissues are upset then serious consequences can result. For example, a fall in blood pressure may reduce the hydrostatic pressure to such an extent that it is incapable of overpowering the opposing protein osmotic pressure, so that the tissue cells are not perfused and become damaged due to lack of oxygen and nutrients. Therefore, to maintain life there must be adequate perfusion which itself depends on the presence of an adequate blood pressure.

On the other hand, at the distal part of the capillary, the hydrostatic pressure may be too great and impede the return of fluid from the tissues. If for example the right side of the heart fails to fully dispose of its pre-load (p.119) then congestion occurs in the great veins, and eventually this back pressure is transmitted further and further back to the capillaries. Such increased hydrostatic pressure prevents some of the fluid being returned to the capillaries, and is therefore retained in the interstitial tissue spaces causing swelling (edema) of the involved limb or organ. Accumulation of fluid in the tissue spaces may compress the tissue cells, preventing the free movement of oxygen to them, and eventually causing cell death due to lack of oxygen.

Disturbances of the osmotic pressure of the plasma proteins can also upset the balance. A shortage of plasma proteins (hypoproteinemia) reduces the osmotic pressure of the plasma so that fluid is left in the tissues, causing swelling of the interstitial spaces, inadequate perfusion and hypoxia of the cells.

Damage to the capillary walls makes them permeable to plasma protein enabling some of it to escape into the tissues. The result is that the effects of the proteins are transferred from the inside to the outside of the capillaries. The fluid, therefore, is pushed into the tissue spaces initially by the greater hydrostatic pressure within the capillaries, but is prevented from returning to the spaces because the osmotic pressure of the escaped protein succeeds in keeping some of it in the tissues. This results in oedema and loss of returning blood volume so that hypotension and collapse can occur.

TISSUE PERFUSION

Adequate tissue perfusion demands:

(1) An adequate hydrostatic pressure at the proximal end of the capillary which itself requires an adequate blood pressure.
(2) An adequate drainage from the distal end of the capillary which depends upon:
  (a) the heart functioning satisfactorily.
  (b) an adequate plasma protein level. This may be lowered by a specific lack of protein within the capillaries, due to malnutrition or excessive infusion of crystalloids, or to an excessive escape of plasma proteins into the tissue spaces due to an increase in permeability of the capillary walls.

Disturbances in circulatory fluids

TRAUMA

Hemorrhage results in the loss of whole blood, a term which includes loss of plasma, red blood cells (RBCs) and other blood cells. Loss of part of the circulatory blood volume is known as hypovolemia, and if uncorrected produces hypotension which is known as hypovolemic hypotension.

Compensatory changes take place in an attempt to maintain the blood pressure:

(1) The circulatory time is reduced, and the heart rate is increased (p. 125).

(2)   The peripheral resistance is increased due to constriction of the arterioles (p. 125) causing pallor.

These are accompanied by sweating, shallow rapid respiration, and sometimes by dilated pupils (p. 126).

If compensation is inadequate the blood pressure falls, and may cause impaired tissue perfusion the effects of which depend on the organs involved; inadequate perfusion of:

> brain causes drowsiness, confusion, coma and death;
> heart causes collapse and death;
> kidney causes reduced (oliguria) or absent (anuria) urine production;
> skin causes pallor.

BURNS

Following a burn injury there is loss of circulating fluid. Although some whole blood is lost due to the destroyed or damaged tissue by far the greatest loss is that of plasma including its protein fraction. Because the plasma loss leaves the RBCs behind there is a reduction in circulating fluid and what is left shows an increased concentration of cells, that is there is hemoconcentration.

The outcome is the same as occurs following hemorrhage, namely tachycardia, eventual hypotension and death, unless the plasma deficiency is made good by plasma infusion.

VOMITING AND/OR DIARRHEA

Total body fluid content = intracellular fluid + extracellular fluid
(interstitial fluid + intravascular fluid)

The fluid inside the cells (intracellular fluid) and that between the cells (interstitial fluid) are available to replenish the circulating fluid (intravascular fluid) and vice versa.

Therefore, if severe vomiting or diarrhea persists, or if fluids and electrolytes such as sodium and chloride are lost through fistulae, the loss of fluid from the interstitial compartment of the extracellular fluid is made up from the intracellular fluid. However, the cells can survive a loss of only a certain amount of their water and electrolyte content, and eventually any further loss of fluid to the exterior can only be compensated for at the expense of the intravascular fluid. The effect of loss of fluid from the interstitial and intracellular compartments results in the symptoms and signs of dehydration, e.g. thirst, lethargy, a dry inelastic skin, sunken eyes (sunken fontanelles in a baby), a dry and dirty tongue, and oliguria or anuria. Loss of intravascular fluid causes tachycardia, hypotension and eventually collapse and coma. These patients respond best to the replacement of the fluid and electrolytes they have lost. Usually they need water and salt, so an infusion of several litres of normal saline (p. 137) may result in a rapid and dramatic improvement.

CHOICE OF INFUSION AGENTS
The type of agent transfused depends on the type of fluid loss.

If RBCs and plasma are lost give whole blood
If plasma is lost give plasma or a plasma substitute (p. 136)
If RBCs are deficient give packed cells
If water and electrolytes are lost give saline.

Whole blood
This has two main functions. First, to maintain the circulating blood volume and, second, to carry oxygen in its cells to the tissues. Provided the blood volume is maintained the tissues still remain adequately oxygenated even if the number of RBCs is reduced by half, giving a hemoglobin in the male, of 8 g per 100 ml. Because tissue perfusion is of paramount importance, if whole blood is unavailable, plasma, plasma substitute (p.136), or crystalloid solutions such as 0.9% saline (normal saline) or Hartmann's solution must be infused as a temporary measure. However, it must be appreciated that if blood loss continues, and the plasma or plasma substitute or crystalloid infusion is not replaced by whole blood, there comes a time when the concentration of the existing RBCs in the cardiovascular system becomes so diluted that their reduced oxygen-carrying capacity falls below that necessary to provide adequate tissue oxygenation; the patient then becomes hypoxic.

Infusions of crystalloid solutions are less effective in the treatment of hemorrhage than are plasma and plasma substitutes. This is because they contain no protein and very quickly pass through the capillary walls and remain in the tissues as interstitial fluid. Therefore, besides having no oxygen-carrying power, due to the absence of RBCs, they are also ineffective in maintaining the circulatory fluid volume for more than a short time (¼–1 hour). They are, however, used in an emergency situation whilst the patient is awaiting the arrival of more suitable infusions.

Packed cells
Hypoxia is the great danger in anemia, due to decreased oxygen-carrying power resulting from the decreased number of RBCs. Usually however the circulating blood volume is normal, and treatment consists

of restoring the oxygen-carrying power by giving RBCs. These can be infused as whole blood, but the plasma fraction increases the circulating blood volume which may cause additional stress on a distressed heart. Therefore, to avoid unnecessary cardiac work the most suitable infusion agent consists of 'packed cells' produced from whole blood by removing some of its plasma and other cells in the laboratory. 'Packed cells' have a higher concentration of RBCs but a lower plasma content than an equal volume of whole blood.

Plasma

Plasma is used for the treatment of burns, peritonitis, septic shock and in hypoproteinemia. Because it has little oxygen-carrying capacity due to the absence of RBCs it is not the first choice in the treatment of hemorrhage. It is available in two forms.

(1) Dry pooled plasma. This needs reconstituting with sterile water. 'Pooled' means that the plasma is taken from a quantity or pool of plasma provided by ten different donors. Theoretically, it has ten times more chance of infecting the recipient with a transmissable disease such as serum hepatitis than has a transfusion of whole blood. In practice transmission of disease is now rare because in most countries blood donations are checked for serum hepatitis and so the risk of its transmission is low. Dry pooled plasma is rapidly becoming obsolete in the UK and is being replaced by plasma protein fraction.

(2) Plasma protein fraction (PPF). This has a much more limited shelf-life. It is very expensive because 4–5 donations of blood are needed to provide 400 ml PPF. It has an advantage in that it does not transmit serum hepatitis.

Plasma substitutes

These are used either when plasma is unavailable or because they are preferred. The one most used is dextran.

Dextran is a polymerized polysaccharide. 'Polysaccharide' means a complex carbohydrate molecule and 'polymerized' signifies that a group of the molecules are stuck together without altering their individual composition.

Dextran is available as dextran 40, 70 and 110. These numbers refer to their molecular weights. For example, dextran 40 has an average molecular weight of 40 000, dextran 70 has a molecular weight of 70 000 and so on. They are available dissolved in dextrose or saline. The higher the molecular weight the longer they stay in the circulation. Dextran 40, 70 and 110 remain in the circulation for 4–6 h, 6–12 h, and 12 h or more respectively, before being excreted via the kidneys.

They retain fluid in the cardiovascular system because their component molecules exert an osmotic pressure (p. 131) similar to that of the plasma proteins.

Dextran 110 interferes with blood cross-matching techniques and so a sample of blood for cross-matching should be taken before dextran 110 is introduced into the circulation.

Dextran can be used whenever plasma is indicated to restore the circulating blood volume. The volume transfused should be restricted to 1 litre because it reduces the clotting factors found in plasma. It is supposed to prevent sludging of corpuscles in the vessels and thus helps to prevent thrombosis occurring as a result of injury, operation or stasis. It cannot transmit serum hepatitis.

Normal saline 0.9% is given in the Accident and Emergency department in cases of blood or plasma loss as a 'starter' whilst awaiting the arrival of more suitable agents, or whenever the main disturbance is loss of salt (p. 134) and water.

0.18% saline with 4% dextrose, 5% dextrose, or Hartmann's solution are given as starters or in cases of dehydration.

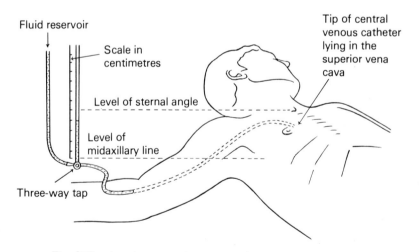

The CVP value above may be expressed as
  − 1 cmH$_2$O pressure with respect to the sternal angle
or + 4 cmH$_2$O pressure with respect to the midaxillary line

Figure 15.2

RATE OF INFUSION

The rate of infusion depends on the clinical condition. A close watch is kept on the pulse rate, the blood pressure and the state of the neck veins. Improvement in the circulating blood volume is accompanied by a decrease in pulse rate and an increase in blood pressure. As the patient improves further there is increased perfusion of the skin which becomes warmer and less pale. The conscious patient may become less anxious and the comatose patient may waken.

Although the above clinical signs are frequently used whenever large volumes of fluid need to be transfused, it is advisable to set up a central venous pressure (CVP) line (Figure 15.2). This consists of a cannula introduced via an arm vein and directed until its tip lies in the superior vena cava (SVC). Its proximal end is connected to a ⊥ piece, the upright part of which is attached to a scale which records the pressure in the tubing and therefore in the SVC. It is important to level and maintain the zero marking of the scale at a point opposite the right atrium. This is obtained by placing the zero mark at the junction of the front third and middle third of the chest or about 2.5 cm (1 inch) below (posterior to) the anterior fold of the axilla.

Function of central venous pressure (CVP) line

During spontaneous inspiration the walls of the SVC are sucked outwards and the pressure within the SVC falls. During spontaneous expiration the intrathoracic pressure increases and is transmitted to the walls of the SVC. Therefore, its walls are compressed and its contents squeezed so that the SVC pressure rises. Hence, the pressure in the SVC (also referred to as the CVP pressure) fluctuates, and so therefore does the fluid in the CVP line. If it does not fluctuate, it is faulty, perhaps the hole in its tip is occluded against the vein wall or, less likely, the patient has had a cardiac arrest.

During spontaneous respiration the normal SVC pressure fluctuates from $+2$ to -2 cmH$_2$O. Loss of circulating fluid causes the CVP to fall if compensatory vasoconstriction (p. 134) does not occur or is inadequate. If fluids are infused at a greater rate than they are being lost and blood volume is restored, the CVP pressure gradually rises to normal. If the CVP pressure rises above normal then the infusion has exceeded what was required.

Sometimes it is difficult for a doctor, when confronted by a shocked patient with a diseased heart, to know whether the heart has the ability to deal with an infusion. In these circumstances a rapid infusion may cause heart failure. This problem may be overcome by trying the effect of a small increment of infusion fluid. The technique is to inject, intravenously, 300 ml of fluid quickly. If the heart can cope with this pre-load and discharge it into the arterial side of the circulation the CVP does not rise above normal. It is then concluded that the heart is capable of dealing with larger volumes of fluid and that transfusion can proceed. If, however, the heart cannot dispose of this 300 ml pre-load the CVP rises above normal and it is obvious that the heart cannot cope well with larger volumes and that infusion must proceed with care.

Shock

Shock may be defined as an inadequate perfusion of the tissues which is severe enough to lead to cellular damage.

Four main types are recognized:

(1) Hypovolemic (hemorrhagic)
(2) Septicemic, bacteremic, or endotoxic
(3) Cardiogenic
(4) Anaphylactic.

HYPOVOLEMIC SHOCK (HEMORRHAGIC)

A decrease in the circulating blood volume due to hemorrhage causes tachycardia, hypotension, sweating and pallor. The treatment is to stop the bleeding and, if necessary, infuse the patient with whole blood, plasma or plasma substitute.

The administration of oxygen does little to improve the situation because of the lack of oxygen carrying RBCs.

Unless bleeding is from the head it is advisable to tilt the patient slightly head down to improve the venous return to the heart, which in turn is then more able to help maintain the blood pressure. However, care is necessary in the obese or pregnant patient whose abdominal contents may impede the movements of the diaphragm, and cause respiratory distress. Pulmonary or cardiac disease may also cause respiratory embarrassment if the patient is placed in the head-down position.

SEPTICEMIC SHOCK

This is due to infection and usually follows abdominal conditions such as peritonitis following a perforated bowel, appendicitis or septic abortion. It can, however, be caused by urinary catheterization. Although it presents in many forms, usually with a pyrexia, there may be hypotension but with a warm, pink skin showing that the arterioles are dilated. Such a state is known as 'warm hypotension'. The arteriolar dilatation is due to the liberation of potentially toxic vasodilator substances such as histamine and kinins.

The role of the Accident and Emergency nurse in this type of shock is to prepare for intravenous infusion (p. 135) and for the administration of antibiotics.

CARDIOGENIC SHOCK

Coronary occlusion leads to impaired cardiac function and often provokes the onset of cardiac irregularities. Emergency treatment consists of reducing the amount of work done by the heart, the patient being allowed to rest in the position which he finds the most comfortable. Pain is relieved by the administration of morphine, diamorphine or Entonox (p. 231). Oxygen should also be given to improve myocardial oxygenation. Intravenous infusion, drug therapy and possible defibrillation depend on the condition of the individual patient.

ANAPHYLACTIC SHOCK

Reaction to foreign proteins is usually accompanied by rashes, intolerable itching of the face, palms, soles of the feet or the anus. Later there may be swelling of the lips, tongue and larynx causing respiratory obstruction. Fortunately deaths are rare but respiratory obstruction may call for urgent endotracheal intubation (see Table 18.1, p. 183), tracheal puncture with a wide bore needle or intravenous cannula (p. 188), or the performance of a tracheostomy (p. 188). Subcutaneous adrenaline (epinephrine) 1 ml of a 1 in 1000 solution at the rate of 0.1–0.2 ml/min is advocated, followed by intravenous hydrocortisone succinate 100 mg, and chlorpheniramine maleate 10–20 mg given by slow intravenous injection.

NEUROGENIC OR VASOVAGAL 'SHOCK'

Tissue damage is unlikely and so this condition, where the patient suddenly loses consciousness due to grief or pain, is not regarded as true shock as defined on p. 139. Recovery is usually rapid if the head is lowered or the legs are raised.

16

Respiratory physiology

F. WILSON

Resuscitation plays an important part in Accident and Emergency care. Often the nurse is the first person to meet and treat the emergency admission. Skill in resuscitative measures such as the relief of respiratory obstruction, the administration of oxygen and the performance of artificial ventilation often proves to be life saving.

However, before resuscitation techniques are discussed it is necessary for the nurse to understand the meaning of such terms as tidal volume, dead space and effective tidal volume (alveolar ventilation). Familiarity with their use also leads to a better understanding of the symptoms, signs and the treatment of a variety of conditions both medical and surgical, encountered in the Accident and Emergency department.

Nevertheless, definitions themselves can cause misunderstanding unless it is realised that the 'barriers' which separate the different volumes of air in the respiratory tract are imaginary. For example, the dead space air (p. 151) consists of that air situated in the nose, mouth, pharynx, larynx, trachea, bronchi and bronchioles, whereas the alveolar air is that air which exists within the alveoli. These descriptions suggest that the dead space air and alveolar air are distinctly separate volumes of air. Their definition creates an artificial barrier between them. In actual fact there is no barrier and mixing of these two 'pockets' of air is a continuous process similar to that seen in a room when a person gently puffs out a cloud of tobacco smoke which intermingles quickly and thoroughly with the surrounding atmosphere. Therefore, in spite of our definitions there is always some mixing between adjoining volumes of air such as the alveolar air and the dead space air even when the patient holds his breath.

Tidal volume
If the nurse finds difficulty in understanding movements of air she should imagine that something visible such as water is breathed in and out of the lungs. At once the significance of the term 'tidal volume'

141

becomes more obvious, particularly if she recalls the tidal movements of the sea around our coasts, for as the sea flows in and ebbs out of the bays so the air moves in and out of the chest during a normal respiration. Just as the quantity of water which leaves the bay during the ebb is approximately equal to the volume of water which entered during the flood so during respiration is the volume of air expired equal to the volume of air inspired. Therefore, the tidal volume of water can be defined as the volume of water which flows either in or out during a normal tide. It is then easy to appreciate why the tidal volume of air is defined as that volume of air which is breathed in or out during a single quiet respiration.

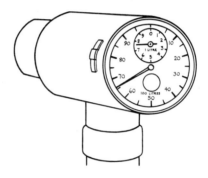

Figure 16.1   Wright's respirometer for measurement of tidal volume

MEASUREMENT OF TIDAL VOLUME
Tidal volume is measured on the Wright's respirometer (Figure 16.1). The co-operative conscious patient places the end of the respirometer in his mouth, nips his nose between finger and thumb, and breathes quietly. The volume of air expired or inspired through the respirometer is recorded on the dial.

   If the patient is unco-operative or cannot co-operate the respirometer is attached to a face mask which is then applied over the patient's mouth and nose. Firm application is necessary to prevent leakage, otherwise false readings will result.

   In the intubated patient the respirometer is connected to the endotracheal connector and endotracheal tube by means of a piece of rubber tubing and a catheter mount (see p. 226).

NORMAL TIDAL VOLUME
The tidal volume of a normal adult varies between 300 and 500 ml, according to such factors as the size of the chest, whether the patient

smokes heavily, or is a trained athlete. Much smaller values are recorded in children, the premature newborn baby often having a tidal volume of only 10 ml.

Tidal volume is symbolized V_T where V = volume
$$T = tidal$$

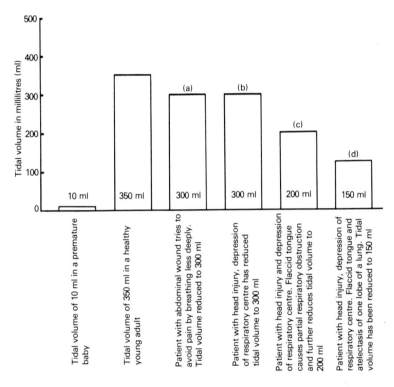

Figure 16.2   Factors affecting tidal volume

REDUCTION OF TIDAL VOLUME (Figure 16.2)

(1) *Obstructive lesions*

The normal tidal volume is reduced by any source of obstruction within the respiratory tract. The commonest cause of partial respiratory obstruction in the unconscious patient is failure to support the lower jaw. In such circumstances the flaccid tongue restricts the flow of air to and from the lungs and thereby diminishes the tidal volume.

Complete respiratory obstruction reduces the tidal volume to zero and death can occur within 30–90 seconds despite vigorous attempts by the respiratory muscles to procure the entry of fresh air into the lungs.

(2) *Non-obstructive lesions*

Non-obstructive lesions can also reduce the tidal volume. Pain following rib fracture or pleurisy causes the patient to restrict movements of the chest wall. This splintage diminishes the tidal excursions and prevents coughing, so that retention of sputum may reduce the effectiveness of his tidal volume (p. 158). Similarly, abdominal pain due to injury, peritonitis or the perforation of a gastric or duodenal ulcer encourages the patient to immobilize his wound by diminishing the movement of his diaphragm.

Reduction in depth of respiration follows overdosage of sedatives and most analgesics or may be due to weakness of the respiratory muscles in poliomyelitis or the Guillain–Barré syndrome (p. 269).

Head injury may cause a reduction in tidal volume and usually does so as a result of a combination of a depressed respiratory centre, due to increased intracranial pressure, the relaxed tongue and accumulation of secretions.

MINUTE VOLUME

Assessment of ventilation demands not only a measurement of the tidal volume but also knowledge of the rate of respiration. Consequently minute volume is defined as the total amount of air which is breathed in or out in 1 minute.

Its value is obtained by adding together all the tidal volumes which the patient breathes in 1 minute. Provided all the tidal volumes are of equal value, say 400 ml, and the patient breathes ten times every minute then the minute volume is 400×10 ml $= 4.0$ litres.

From this reasoning the mathematician or the physiologist quotes the definition in a more concise way and says minute volume $=$ average tidal volume $\times$ number of respirations per minute.

An electrical version of the Wright's respirometer is now available which gives a direct readout of the minute volume on a scale, relieving the nurse of all the calculations.

The minute volume may be reduced by any condition which causes a reduction in either the tidal volume or the respiratory rate or both.

Minute volume is symbolized $\dot{V}_T$

where:

$V =$ volume

$\cdot$ signifies that time is involved, usually a period of 1 minute.

Therefore $\dot{V}$ $=$ volume per minute

$\qquad V_T =$ tidal volume

Therefore $\dot{V}_T =$ tidal volume per minute

which is rewritten

$\qquad \dot{V}_T =$ minute volume

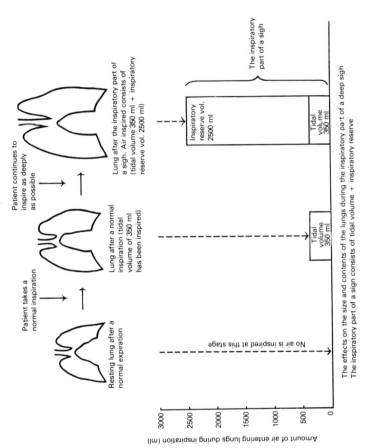

Figure 16.3 Effect of sigh – inspiration

The 'sigh'

INSPIRATORY RESERVE VOLUME

Healthy patients who are observed whilst relaxing, sleeping, working or eating demonstrate that there are many normal deviations from the standard respiratory pattern of regular quiet respiration. A frequent variation is the sigh which can be defined as the audible manifestation of a prolonged inspiration followed by a prolonged expiration. It is obvious that during the inspiratory part of a sigh a greater volume of air than the tidal volume is inspired (Figure 16.3). In other words, when the tidal volume has entered the lungs, further inspiratory effect results in more air being breathed in. This extra lung capacity may be regarded as being 'in reserve' for whenever the occasion requires the patient to take in a deep breath. The proper term for this particular part of the lung volume is the inspiratory reserve volume which is defined as the maximal volume of air that can be inspired after completing a normal inspiration. Normal values of the inspiratory reserve volume are 2000–3200 ml (2.0–3.2 l). The patient makes use of his inspiratory reserve volume and his expiratory reserve volume (see below) when he takes deep breaths in an attempt to maintain the normal blood gas tensions (p. 232) and pH (p. 245) of his blood or restore them to within acceptable limits.

EXPIRATORY RESERVE VOLUME

The expiratory part of the sigh (Figure 16.4) is particularly noticeable in circumstances of great sadness, weariness or relief, when the expiratory phase is prolonged and an additional quantity of air is forced out of the lungs. The volume of this additional or reserve air, which is available for expulsion from the lungs during a forced expiration, is known as the expiratory reserve volume and is defined as the maximal volume of air which can be expressed after a normal tidal expiration.

The presence of the expiratory reserve volume and the residual volume (p. 148) enables interchange of gases between lungs and blood to continue should the patient hold his breath for any reason after a normal expiration. It also explains why he is able to survive for some time even when respiratory obstruction occurs immediately after an expiration. Normal values of the expiratory reserve volume are 750–1000 ml (0.75–1.0 l).

Vital capacity

The values of tidal volume, inspiratory reserve volume and expiratory reserve volume, when added together, constitute the vital capacity (Figures 16.3–16.6) which is defined as the maximal volume of air that can be expelled from the lungs by a forceful effort after a maximal

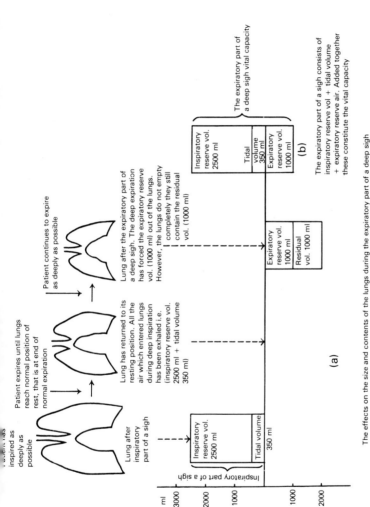

The effects on the size and contents of the lungs during the expiratory part of a deep sigh

Figure 16.4 Effect of sigh – expiration

inspiration. This is easily understood when it is remembered that a maximal inspiration draws into the lungs a volume equal to the tidal volume plus the inspiratory reserve volume. Then, in a forced expiration, following the maximal inspiration, the inspiratory reserve volume and tidal volume are expelled first but as expiration continues the expiratory reserve volume is also expelled into the surrounding atmosphere.

Vital capacity is reduced by anything that interferes with the movement of the lungs, chest wall or diaphragm. The presence of air or blood in the pleural cavity, infection of lung tissue and abdominal distension due to obesity, gas, ascites or tumour all reduce the vital capacity and cause breathlessness on exertion or even at rest.

Vital capacity varies between 3000–5000 ml (3.0–5.0 l).

In gross abdominal distension, or severe lung disease, the vital capacity may be reduced to as little as 500 ml, i.e. the tidal volume of a healthy adult patient. He is then unable to improve his ventilation by taking the deep breaths necessary for physical effort, such as walking up stairs or for restoring to normal a raised blood carbon dioxide concentration (p. 238) caused by pulmonary infection. Very soon his carbon dioxide tension (p. 235) becomes so high that he loses consciousness and dies, unless his carbon dioxide narcosis (p. 243) is treated.

Residual volume
Even though a forced expiration expels the expiratory reserve air, the lungs do not empty completely. A residual amount of air remains in the lungs. This air, therefore, is termed the residual volume and is described as the volume of air which remains in the lungs after a maximal expir-

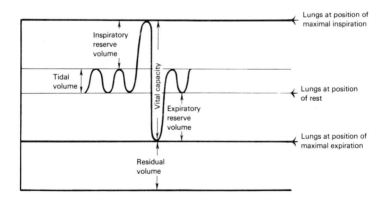

Figure 16.5   Lung volumes

atory effort. The normal residual volume is 1000–1500 ml (1.0–1.5 l).

The residual volume increases as the patient ages, especially if the patient has obvious obstructive small airway disease such as emphysema or asthma. In both conditions the patient has progressive difficulty in emptying the lungs as fully as a normal patient until eventually he is unable to do so. Incomplete emptying of the lungs then leaves behind an additional residue of air and so the residual volume increases.

All the above volumes are also illustrated in Figure 16.5.

TRAPPING

Because some of the air prevented from leaving the chest is trapped, the process described above is appropriately called trapping. It partly accounts for the inability of the middle-aged man to run as fast as his children. He is unable to get enough air out of his chest fast enough during the time his strenuous efforts allow him for expiration. He therefore becomes breathless (dyspneic).

Any infection which causes swelling of the mucous membranes and narrowing of the air passages has a greater effect on this type of person, so that even at rest breathlessness may become pronounced.

Alveolar air

Although the respiratory tract consists of the mouth and nose, oropharynx and nasopharynx, larynx, trachea, bronchi, bronchioles and alveoli, it is only the walls of the alveoli that are especially adapted to allow gases to pass through them to enter or leave the blood in the pulmonary capillaries, so that the interchange of oxygen and carbon dioxide with the blood is restricted to the air which is present in the alveolar spaces. This air, within the alveoli, is termed the alveolar air and in a healthy adult at the end of a quiet expiration amounts to about 2500 ml (2.5 l). Smaller values are found if the alveoli contain sputum or edema fluid.

Due to the movements of the respiratory muscles, the beating of the heart and the muscular activity of the patient, the air within the alveoli is in a state of permanent agitation even during the expiratory pause (see below). Such alveolar air movement enables continuous replenishment of the oxygen to, and removal of the carbon dioxide from, the immediate vicinity of the blood vessels within the alveolar walls.

In health the interchange of gases between the alveolar air and blood in the pulmonary capillaries is extremely efficient. Within the 0.75 seconds which a blood corpuscle takes to traverse a pulmonary capillary it is depleted of its unwanted carbon dioxide and is almost fully oxygenated in return.

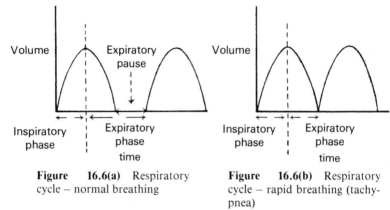

Figure 16.6(a) Respiratory cycle – normal breathing

Figure 16.6(b) Respiratory cycle – rapid breathing (tachypnea)

The phases of respiration

The stages of a normal respiratory cycle are illustrated by any resting healthy adult (Figure 16.6a and b). He inspires, immediately expires and then pauses for a short time before he breathes again.

The inspiratory part of the cycle is called the *inspiratory phase* which lasts from the beginning of inspiration to the end of the same inspiration.

The *expiratory phase* occupies the rest of the cycle and consists of the period during which the lungs deflate combined with an interval or rest period that is termed the *expiratory pause* which exists between the end of deflation and the start of the next inflation.

The mixing of gases within the lungs and their interchange between the alveoli and the blood vessels takes place continuously throughout all stages of the respiratory cycle. As a result, during expiration, and during the expiratory pause, the oxygen concentration in the alveoli and blood falls and the carbon dioxide level rises.

The consequent and varying carbon dioxide levels in the alveoli and the blood change the respiratory pattern because carbon dioxide is the main stimulus to respiration. A raised blood carbon dioxide concentration stimulates the respiratory centre in the brain and increases the rate and depth of respiration. If the level of carbon dioxide in the body falls the reverse happens and the rate and depth of respiration decrease.

The Accident and Emergency nurse should be familiar with the different phases of respiration because they are important when she performs intermittent positive pressure ventilation (p. 221) by means of a resuscitation bag (p. 222) or a mechanical ventilator (p. 223).

During exertion, or with infection of the lungs, the expiratory pause is not seen (Figure 16.6b) because the urgent need to maintain an increased respiratory exchange allows no time for a rest period, since the carbon dioxide level rises more quickly than when the patient is at rest and in good health. In such circumstances the expiratory phase consists only of the time taken for lung deflation.

ANATOMICAL DEAD SPACE – DEAD SPACE AIR

Because that part of the respiratory tract extending from the mouth and nose down to and including the bronchioles does not come into intimate contact with the pulmonary capillaries it can be regarded as non-existent or functionally 'dead' as far as actual gaseous exchange with the blood is concerned. In consequence, the space within is described as the dead space, and the dead space air is defined as that volume of air within the respiratory tract which does not partake in respiratory exchange.

Although dead space varies with the individual, a fairly reliable value can be obtained if the weight of the person is known. For most purposes the dead space is regarded as being 2 ml for every 1 kg (1 ml/lb) body weight.

i.e. if weight is 5 kg (10 lb) the dead space is 10 ml;
if weight is 70 kg (140 lb) the dead space is 140 ml;*
Dead space volume is symbolized V_D
V = volume
D = dead space.

The significance of the dead space in health and disease is discussed below.

AIR MOVEMENTS BETWEEN ATMOSPHERE, DEAD SPACE AND ALVEOLAR AIR

Inspiration and the effective tidal volume

Because of the dead space in the respiratory tract it is clear that all the air which enters the nose and mouth when the patient inspires does not enter the lungs. On inspiration the first air to enter the lungs and mix with the alveolar air is the dead space air which is already present within that part of the respiratory tract extending from the bronchioles to the nose and mouth. Therefore, the 'bronchiolar' and 'bronchial' air pass into the alveoli. †At the same time the 'laryngeal' and 'tracheal air' move into the bronchi and bronchioles. Likewise, fresh air simultaneously moves into the mouth and nose and then passes into the lower parts of the respiratory tract, whereupon some of it reaches the alveoli. To summarize these events, two main changes can be regarded as taking

*These figures are only approximate because 1 kg = 2.2 lb.
. †In physiology the dead space is never subdivided into 'bronchial, tracheal, laryngeal' air etc. These subdivisions of the tidal air are invented to help clarify the terms 'effective tidal volume' and 'alveolar ventilation'.

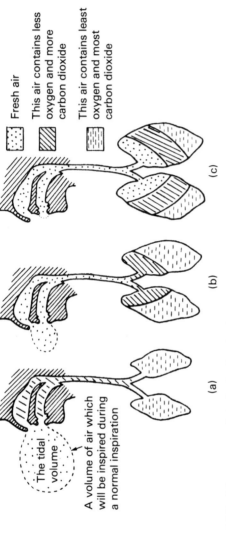

Fresh air

This air contains less oxygen and more carbon dioxide

This air contains least oxygen and most carbon dioxide

The tidal volume

A volume of air which will be inspired during a normal inspiration

(a)

(b)

(c)

Figure 16.7   Movements of air during inspiration.

(a) During resting stage (after a normal expiration the lungs contain the expiratory reserve volume and the residual volume which together constitute the air in the alveoli, i.e. the alveolar air).

(b) Halfway through inspiration:
    (i) Dead space air has entered lungs.
    (ii) Fresh air has filled dead space.

(c) At end of inspiration lungs contain:
    (i) Old expiratory reserve volume and residual volume.
    (ii) Dead space air.
    (iii) Fresh atmospheric air.

The diagrams imply that the different kinds of air are separate. This is not so. It is important to realize that intimate mixing occurs within the lungs at all stages of the respiratory cycle.

place during inspiration; the dead space air followed by part of the inspired fresh air enters the lungs and mixes with the alveolar air (Figure 16.7a–c) so that the air in the lungs at this stage consists of 'old' alveolar air, dead space air and fresh air. Simultaneously, fresh air fills the dead space. Therefore, only a proportion of the inspired fresh air reaches the lungs and effectively ventilates the alveoli. These events help to explain the term *effective tidal volume* which is described as that part of the tidal volume which enters the alveoli and is available to take part in gaseous exchange with the blood.

The effective tidal volume is equal to the actual tidal volume minus the dead space volume;

i.e. effective tidal volume = tidal volume – dead space volume

∴ if tidal volume = 440 ml
and dead space = 140 ml
then the effective tidal volume = 440 ml – 140 ml = 300 ml.

Because the effective tidal volume is that volume of gas that enters the alveoli it is symbolized V_A.

Therefore, the expression
effective tidal volume = tidal volume – dead space volume
can be written
$$V_A = V_T - V_D$$

Effective minute volume (alveolar ventilation)
The effective minute volume is measured by adding together all the effective tidal volumes which the patient breathes in 1 minute. Provided all the tidal volumes are approximately equal then the effective minute volume = effective tidal volume × number of respirations per minute.

If effective tidal volume = 300 ml
and respiratory rate = 12 per minute
then effective minute volume = 300 × 12
= 3600 ml = 3.6 l.

Because the effective minute volume is that volume which ventilates the alveoli, the effective minute volume is usually referred to as the alveolar ventilation and is symbolized in physiology books as $\dot{V}_A$.

V = volume. The dot · above the V signifies that the volume is measured over a period of time, usually a minute.

Therefore, $\dot{V}$ = volume per minute
         A = alveolar
Therefore, $\dot{V}_A$ = alveolar ventilation per minute.

Therefore
$$\dot{V}_A = \dot{V}_T - \dot{V}_D$$

Alveolar ventilation per minute	=	all the tidal volumes added together over a period of one minute, that is the minute volume.	$-$	the dead space volume	$\times$	the number of breaths taken during one minute.

EXPIRATION

On expiration, the deflating lungs squeeze some of the stale air from the alveoli into the dead space (Figure 16.8a–d). As a result all the fresh air existing in the dead space at the end of the previous inspiration is forced out of the mouth and nose and is returned to the atmosphere without ever entering the lungs. Immediately after this, as expiration continues, part of the stale alveolar air (p. 151) is also expelled and its carbon dioxide is rapidly lost to the surrounding atmosphere.

At the end of expiration the dead space contains only air which has been squeezed out of the lungs and which must contain less oxygen and more carbon dioxide than fresh atmospheric air because it has already taken part in gaseous exchange with the pulmonary capillaries. At the beginning of the next respiratory cycle, as indicated by the onset of inspiration, no fresh air can reach the alveoli until the used dead space air has first entered the lungs and mixed with the alveolar air (Figure 16.7a–c).

Therefore, if the tidal volume is diminished until it equals or is less than the dead space volume only the dead space air reaches the alveoli so causing a fatal degree of oxygen lack and carbon dioxide excess (p. 160). Such severe respiratory embarrassment due to hypoventilation can occur suddenly, but a more frequent occurrence is where the patient's condition shows slight respiratory insufficiency which gradually deteriorates into respiratory failure (p. 239). In such circumstances, where ventilation of the alveoli is reduced the patient is said to be hypoventilating and needs urgent treatment, usually by means of bag and mask (p. 222).

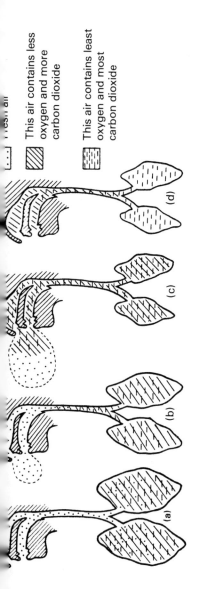

This air contains less oxygen and more carbon dioxide

This air contains least oxygen and most carbon dioxide

Figure 16.8 Movements of air during expiration

(a) At start of expiration lungs contain air which has given up part of its oxygen to the blood and in return has received carbon dioxide from the blood. It can be regarded as stale air.

(b) Halfway through expiration:

  (i) The unaltered fresh air in the dead space is breathed out without ever entering lung.

  (ii) Some of stale air has moved out into the dead space.

(c) At the end of expiration:

  (i) Some stale air is expelled from nose and mouth.

  (ii) Dead space contains stale air.

  (iii) Some stale air remains in lungs.

(d) (i) During expiratory pause (between end of expiration and start of next inspiration) gaseous exchange still occurs in lungs.

  (ii) Air remaining in alveoli (alveolar air) becomes more stale with a decreasing amount of oxygen and an increasing amount of carbon dioxide until another inspiration washes out the alveoli again (see Figure 16.7)

The diagrams imply that the different kinds of air are separate. This is not so. It is important to realize that intimate mixing occurs within the lungs at all stages of the respiratory cycle.

Hypoventilation
Underventilation (hypoventilation) of the alveoli is caused by a variety of conditions which can basically be divided into two main groups:

(1) Where the airways are normal but there is injury or depression of:
  (a) The respiratory centre (head injury, overdosage of sedative or narcotic drugs).
  (b) The spinal cord (broken neck or back).
  (c) The peripheral nerves passing from the spinal cord to the diaphragm and intercostal muscles (trauma and Guillain–Barré syndrome p. 269).
  (d) The neuromuscular junction which exists between the ends of the nerve fibres and the voluntary muscles on which they act (myasthenia gravis (p. 269) or muscle relaxants such as d-tubocurarine chloride, pancuronium, gallamine and suxamethonium).
  (e) The chest wall (trauma).

(2) Where the calibre of the airways is reduced, causing respiratory obstruction. Narrowing is caused by:
  (a) The relaxed tongue (coma or anesthesia).
  (b) Secretions (infection or poisonous gas).
  (c) Edema of the mucous membrane (infection or poisonous gas).
  (d) Hypertrophy of the musculature of the bronchi and bronchioles (asthma).

Respiratory embarrassment due to hypoventilation can therefore be caused by many medical and surgical conditions, and although it can occur suddenly its course is usually insidious, and unless carefully observed the patient showing slight respiratory insufficiency may slide gradually into respiratory failure (p. 239). Perhaps the best way to illustrate a typical series of events leading to respiratory insufficiency and respiratory failure is to follow the course of an imaginary patient (Tables 16.1–16.8) with broken ribs who later develops a chest infection. For example:

Table 16.1 represents a healthy patient, before injury occurred, weighing 70 kg (150 lb) whose dead space is 150 ml. His normal chest movements move a tidal volume of 450 ml. His respiratory rate is 10 breaths/minute.

Table 16.1

Tidal volume (ml)	450
Dead space (ml)	150
Effective tidal volume (ml)	300
Respiratory rate per minute	10
Effective minute volume (ml)	$\overline{300 \times 10}$
(alveolar ventilation) =	3000 ml
=	3.0 l

Therefore, the effective tidal volume is 300 ml × 10 = 3000 ml = 3.0 l. He is well oxygenated and he expels his carbon dioxide effectively.

Table 16.2 represents the same patient the day after sustaining two fractured ribs.

Table 16.2

Tidal volume (ml)	300
Dead space (ml)	150
Effective tidal volume (ml)	150
Respiratory rate per minute	10
Effective minute volume (l)	$\overline{150 \times 10}$
(alveolar ventilation) =	1500 ml
=	1.5 l

The dead space remains the same but pain reduces his tidal volume from 450 ml to 300 ml, that is to two-thirds of the original volume.

i.e. new tidal volume = $450 \times \dfrac{2}{3} = \dfrac{900}{3} = 300$ ml

However the effective tidal volume and the effective minute volume are reduced by much more, in fact to half the value existing before the injury occurred.

i.e. effective tidal volume = 300 ml − 150 ml = 150 ml

Therefore, if the respiratory rate were maintained at the original 10 breaths/minute the effective tidal volume would be 150 ml × 10 = 1.5 l, which is half the effective minute volume existing before the injury but because the alveolar ventilation is diminished carbon dioxide begins to accumulate in the alveoli and in the blood. This hypercarbia (p. 239) stimulates the respiratory centre to increase the respiratory rate to 20 breaths/minute (Table 16.3) and thereby restores the alveolar ventilation to his normal 3.0 l.

Table 16.3

Tidal volume (ml)	300
Dead space (ml)	150
Effective tidal volume (ml)	150
Respiratory rate per minute	20
Effective minute volume (ml)	150 × 20
(alveolar ventilation) =	3000 ml
=	3.0 l

Table 16.4 represents the same patient 3 days after injury. Inability to cough up sputum has caused collapse of segments of his lung. Impaired air entry into the lung due to the combination of atelectasis and pain reduces the tidal volume further to 250 ml.

Table 16.4

Tidal volume (ml)	250
Dead space (ml)	150
Effective tidal volume (ml)	100
Respiratory rate per minute	20
Effective minute volume (ml)	100 × 20
(alveolar ventilation) =	2000 ml
=	2.0 l

The effective tidal volume is 250 ml – 150 ml = 100 ml. Similarly, the alveolar ventilation falls to 100 ml × 20 = 2000 ml (2.0 l) unless he is able to increase his rate of respiration. This effective tidal volume of 100 ml may still be adequate to provide sufficient oxygen (p. 239), but the increase in carbon dioxide is not tolerated and so the ventilation has to be improved. He is unable to increase the depth of respiration because of pain and once more increases his respiratory rate, this time to 30 breaths/minute (Table 16.5).

Table 16.5

Tidal volume (ml)	250
Dead space (ml)	150
Effective tidal volume (ml)	100
Respiratory rate per minute	30
Effective minute volume (ml)	100 × 30
(alveolar ventilation) =	3000 ml
=	3.0 l

Table 16.5 shows that although the respiratory rate is now treble that before his injury the effective minute volume, that is the alveolar ventilation, is the same. Therefore, a tidal volume of 250 ml has to be moved three times as often to provide the same ventilation as does a tidal volume of 450 ml (see Table 16.1).

Such an increase in the ventilation rate imposes a corresponding increase in muscular effort, so that the very young and the very old in particular rapidly become fatigued and may die from exhaustion caused by the extra muscular work unless the atelectasis is relieved. If the patient does tolerate the increased respiratory rate he soon develops pneumonia, unless the sputum causing the atelectasis is coughed up or is removed by endotracheal or endobronchial suction (p. 190).

The patient under discussion is now unable to clear his bronchi of sputum. Further atelectasis reduces the effective tidal volume to 30 ml (Table 16.6).

Table 16.6

Tidal volume (ml)	180
Dead space (ml)	150
Effective tidal volume (ml)	30
Respiratory rate per minute	20
Effective tidal volume (ml)	30×20
(alveolar ventilation) =	600 ml
=	0.6 l

His physical fatigue renders him unable to maintain his previous high rate of respiration which has fallen to 20 breaths/minute, making the respiratory exchange of gases in the lungs less efficient. Carbon dioxide accumulates in the alveoli so that he has carbon dioxide retention. This causes a similar rise in the carbon dioxide level of the blood, a condition known as hypercarbia, which, if left uncorrected, produces a fall in pH as the blood becomes more acid (p. 247). Because the increased blood acidity is due primarily to respiratory disturbances he is said to have a respiratory acidosis (p. 248).

Simultaneously the excess carbon dioxide retained in the alveoli takes up space which should be occupied by the oxygen in the inspired air. Therefore, the alveoli contain less oxygen than before causing a fall in oxygen uptake by the lungs and the blood. The amount of unsaturated hemoglobin (p. 162) rises and causes cyanosis (p. 162). This combination of oxygen lack and carbon dioxide retention is called asphyxia which becomes more marked as the tidal volume approaches the same value as the dead space when, of course, life cannot exist because the effective tidal volume is virtually nil (Table 16.7).

Table 16.7

Tidal volume (ml)	150
Dead space (ml)	150
Effective tidal volume (ml)	0
Respiratory rate per minute	10
Effective minute volume (ml) (alveolar ventilation) =	10 × 0 0

In such circumstances the respiratory movements have no effect except to move the dead space air in and out of the lungs without any chance of fresh air entering the alveoli. Giving the patient oxygen to breathe will have little if any beneficial effect because it too will be unable to reach the alveoli. What is needed is an unobstructed airway and an increased tidal volume which are usually accomplished by relieving obstruction (p. 166), aspirating secretions (p. 190), removing pain (p. 231), reducing the dead space (p. 188), artificial ventilation (p. 221) and the use of drugs.

From the above it is therefore obvious that a patient who is breathing rapidly and shallowly is ventilating inefficiently and perhaps inadequately. Such a patient should be constantly observed and be regarded as progressing towards respiratory failure and asphyxia.

The Accident and Emergency nurse should be familiar with these two terms; respiratory failure exists if the patient is unable to carry out an adequate respiratory exchange. It is present if the PaO_2 (p. 235) falls to less than 60 mmHg (8 kPa), together with a rise in $PaCO_2$ (p. 235) to more than 50 mmHg (6.5 kPa), or if there is a combination of the two when breathing air. Respiratory failure can occur as a result of hypoventilation, the presence of a shunt (p. 239) or a combination of both.

Asphyxia (p. 163) is a combination of oxygen lack (hypoxia) and carbon dioxide accumulation (p. 163). Asphyxia is an extreme form of respiratory failure and needs instant attention.

Oxygen and carbon dioxide concentrations
If the Accident and Emergency nurse is conversant with the oxygen and carbon dioxide concentrations found in the lungs and in the blood in health and disease, she will be more capable of understanding why emergency resuscitation is started and how the effects of supportive treatment can be assessed.

Table 16.8 shows the approximate contents of oxygen, carbon dioxide and nitrogen in inspired and expired air.

Table 16.8

	Inspired air (atmospheric air)	*Expired air*
Oxygen content	20 parts	15 parts
Carbon dioxide content	0 parts	5 parts
Nitrogen content	80 parts	80 parts

More accurate values of the components of inspired and expired air, together with the constituents of alveolar air are given in Table 16.9. Their relationship with the partial pressures (tensions, p. 232) of the gases in the blood is discussed in Chapter 24.

Table 16.9 Percentage of composition of inspired, alveolar and expired air

	Inspired (%)	*Alveolar* (%)	*Expired* (%)
Oxygen content	20.9	15.0	16.0
Carbon dioxide content	0.04	5.6	4.5
Nitrogen content	79.0	79.0	79.0
Water content	0.06	0.4	0.5

At this stage, however, Table 16.8 is adequate to explain some important aspects of pulmonary exchange.

The air around us, that is normal atmospheric air, consists of approximately 80 parts nitrogen and 20 parts oxygen (Table 16.8). When the fresh inspired air enters the lungs and comes into contact with the thin linings of the blood vessels in the alveolar walls, about one-quarter (5 parts) of the oxygen enters the bloodstream and is carried to the tissues. Therefore, only a proportion of the oxygen is removed from the inspired air. There is more than enough for the immediate needs of the body. Three-quarters (15 parts) of the inspired oxygen return to the atmosphere on expiration.

Fresh inspired air contains almost no carbon dioxide but when it comes into contact with the blood vessels in the lungs it receives a volume of carbon dioxide which is roughly equal to the volume of oxygen which the blood carries away.

Therefore, if insufficient fresh air enters the lungs the patient may or may not become short of oxygen but his blood will definitely contain an excess of carbon dioxide.

The percentage composition (concentration) of these gases in the alveoli determine their partial pressures or tensions in the alveoli and influence their values in the blood (p. 233).

These vary according to the extent of the reduction in the fresh air supply. If the supply of fresh air is moderately reduced by respiratory obstruction then the blood is able to extract the same amount of oxygen from the reduced volume of inspired air. Because the oxygen content of inspired air is more than sufficient to meet normal demands, the patient does not show any immediate significant ill-effects because the oxygen needs of his tissues are still satisfied. He remains pink in color and the rate and depth of respiration may be unchanged. However, unless the respiratory obstruction is relieved the retention of carbon dioxide (hypercarbia) causes an immediate increase in the depth and rate of respiration. This deeper and faster breathing helps to wash out the excess carbon dioxide, and persists until the carbon dioxide has returned to an acceptably normal level. If, for some reason, the patient is unable to increase his ventilation in this way, then the raised level of carbon dioxide in his blood produces certain signs (p. 163) which must be recognized lest the hypercarbia eventually leads to respiratory failure.

When the supply of fresh air to the tissues is further restricted, as occurs in more severe degrees of respiratory obstruction or respiratory depression, the blood takes an additional quantity of oxygen from any inspired air which manages to reach the lungs, but eventually the oxygen supply falls below that demanded by the tissues which become short of oxygen – the patient is hypoxic and cyanosis may be present. However, the presence of cyanosis depends on the severity of the hypoxia and also on the hemoglobin concentration (see below).

CYANOSIS

Cyanosis is due to the presence of chemically reduced hemoglobin, that is hemoglobin which is not fully oxygenated.

A normal male adult has 15 g hemoglobin in 100 ml blood, approximately 13.7 g/100 ml in the female, which is fully oxygenated on leaving the lungs. If for any reason the hemoglobin is not fully oxygenated as oxyhemoglobin it follows that the remainder must be sub-oxygenated and circulating as reduced hemoglobin. Should the total amount of reduced hemoglobin be 5 g/100 ml (5 g/dl) or more the patient becomes cyanosed. This particular example would leave the male patient with 15 – 5 g/100 ml (15 – 5 g/dl) oxygenated hemoglobin (oxyhemoglobin) on which to survive.

In polycythemia rubra vera the hemoglobin level is often around 20 g/dl; 5 g/dl of reduced hemoglobin would still leave 20 – 5 = 15 g of oxygenated hemoglobin on which to survive. Cyanosis in this type of patient is therefore less serious than in the patient with 5 g/dl reduced hemoglobin and 10 g/dl oxygenated hemoglobin.

If an anemic patient with a hemoglobin level of 9 g/dl is cyanosed it means that at least 5 g/dl of his 9 g/dl hemoglobin is not oxygenated, so he has a maximum of 4 g/dl of oxyhemoglobin to oxygenate his tissues. He is in a far more desperate state than in the normal or polycythemic patient. If he becomes more anemic so that his hemoglobin falls below 5 g/dl he cannot become cyanosed and his condition may be critical due to oxygen lack without him demonstrating any blueness of his skin or mucous membranes.

Cyanosis is best seen in colored races in the mucous membrane of the inside of the lips and in the tongue. In Caucasians it is also seen where the skin is thin, such as in the nail beds, ears and lips.

Types of cyanosis

Central cyanosis is due to sub-oxygenated blood in the arteries, that is, arterial oxygen desaturation. It is caused by inadequate oxygenation of the blood in the lungs or is due to blood by passing the lungs (see shunts, p. 239). The effect of giving oxygen is discussed on p. 240.

Peripheral cyanosis is due to a high oxygen extraction from blood passing through the peripheral regions of the body. It is due to diminished blood flow in those areas and is seen in cardiac failure and shock. It is also frequent in healthy people in cold weather when it soon disappears on warming or rubbing the affected part.

ASPHYXIA

Asphyxia is a combination of oxygen lack and carbon dioxide retention. Asphyxia can occur instantly as a result of an acute respiratory obstruction but then it is usually recognized immediately. Inhalation of stomach contents is a frequent cause of sudden asphyxia.

Gradual asphyxia is harder to detect, but a raised respiratory rate demands very careful observation especially if the patient has a chest infection.

Signs of asphyxia

Asphyxia is likely to be present when the pulse rate and the respiratory rate progressively increase. The volume of the pulse wave is bounding in character and the blood pressure rises by 10–30 mmHg. Beads of perspiration appear on the forehead and in the grooves between the nose and cheeks. The palms become moist, and sweating may be severe enough to soak the bed clothes. When carbon dioxide retention (hypercarbia) is more pronounced than the shortage of oxygen (hypoxia) the patient often has a hot flushed skin. As a consequence of the hot, red, moist skin the hypercarbic patient is often described as having the appearance of a 'sweating lobster'.

As asphyxia becomes more pronounced the mechanisms of the cardiovascular and respiratory systems fail to compensate for the increasing hypoxia and hypercarbia. As a result the pulse becomes weaker in volume, the blood pressure falls, the respirations become more shallow and less frequent and the patient becomes increasingly cyanosed until eventually death occurs.

If some obvious mechanical obstruction is present, in or above the bronchi, the patient makes determined efforts to draw air past the obstruction. Recognition of the signs of obstructed respiration is vital if the patient is to receive appropriate treatment to guarantee his survival.

Relief of asphyxia
Asphyxia is usually relieved by the removal of any factor that interferes with respiratory exchange. In the case of the anesthetized patient, elevation of the chin lifts the obstructing relaxed tongue away from the posterior pharyngeal wall. Aspiration of obstructing secretions through an endotracheal tube or bronchoscope restores the patency of the airway. Ventilation of the lungs of the patient who has received an overdosage of anesthetic or sedative drugs restores the tidal volume towards normal values improving the intake of oxygen and the elimination of carbon dioxide. Relief of asphyxia in these ways is often life saving.

Apart from bronchoscopy all these procedures can be carried out in an emergency by the nurse. Their management is discussed in the appropriate chapters.

17

Respiratory obstruction

F. WILSON

Diagnosis of sudden complete obstruction is simple since the patient becomes cyanosed within a few seconds. Unless relief is immediate the patient dies.

Partial obstruction is equally dangerous because its insidious onset and progress lead to a gradual deterioration of the patient's condition which may remain unrecognized until he collapses and dies. It is important to realize that the presence of an oral airway or endotracheal tube does not guarantee such obstruction will not occur (p. 172).

SIGNS OF RESPIRATORY OBSTRUCTION
The importance of listening to the entry and exit of air from the mouth and nose is described on p. 168. Attention must also be paid to the characteristics of the respiratory movements because they do occur even when complete obstruction is present. The nurse must, therefore, be on her guard to diagnose instantly when these respiratory movements are abnormal. However, before these signs can be appreciated it is necessary to understand the movements involved in normal respiration.

Movements of respiration – normal and obstructed
NORMAL RESPIRATION
The chest muscles and the diaphragm work together to produce respiratory movements. During inspiration the intercostal muscles, which lie between the ribs, contract and pull the ribs outwards. The diaphragm contracts and pushes the abdominal contents downwards. Because the pelvis and vertebrae are rigid structures the extra space required to accommodate the abdominal contents, when they are pressed down by the diaphragm, is obtained by the relaxation and outward movement of the abdominal wall. Therefore, during a normal inspiration the chest wall and the abdominal wall move outwards together and air is drawn into the lungs.

During normal expiration the muscles of the chest wall and the diaphragm relax and together with the normal elasticity of the lungs they force air out of the chest. Acting as one functional unit all these allow the chest and the abdominal wall to move inwards together.

OBSTRUCTED RESPIRATION

When respiratory obstruction is present the muscles of the chest wall and the diaphragm are stimulated to make extra efforts to draw an adequate supply of air into the lungs. Accessory muscles of respiration come to their aid so that the muscles which extend from the neck to the chest also contract during inspiration. Widening of the nostrils may also occur in an attempt to improve the intake of air. At the same time the synchronous movements of the chest and abdominal wall are disturbed because the diaphragm is a much stronger muscle than the combined power of the intercostal and accessory respiratory muscles which surround and pull upon the outside of the chest wall. As a result the diaphragm pulls too hard and overcomes the outward pull of the other muscles so that the chest wall moves inwards during inspiration instead of outwards.

Therefore, during inspiration when respiratory obstruction is present, the chest wall moves inwards and the abdominal wall moves outwards. This type of breathing is called 'reversed' respiration or 'see-saw' respiration.

During expiration the abdominal wall moves inwards as the diaphragm relaxes. The chest wall moves only slightly inwards because during the previous inspiration the excessive pull of the diaphragm has already drawn it inwards to the expiratory position. However, if obstruction is severe the muscles of the abdominal wall may contract very strongly and in their attempt to empty the chest they press the diaphragm into the chest so forcibly that the chest moves outwards.

Prevention and relief of respiratory obstruction

Internal strangulation is an appropriate alternative to the term respiratory obstruction because internal blockage of the respiratory tract is as lethal as tying a rope round the victim's neck. Respiratory obstruction is always harmful. If present it must be relieved. If absent it must be prevented. The two commonest causes of respiratory obstruction and therefore of asphyxia are the relaxed tongue and the inhalation of foreign material such as vomit.

THE RELAXED TONGUE

Respiratory obstruction is most frequently due to the relaxed tongue. On inspection the tongue is seen as a flabby lump of muscle which has

Normal breathing

Inspiration	*Expiration*
Chest wall moves outwards	Chest wall moves inwards
Abdominal wall moves outwards	Abdominal wall moves inwards
Accessory muscles of inspiration are not used	

Obstructed respiration

Inspiration	*Expiration*
Chest wall moves inwards	Chest wall moves inwards but if obstruction is very severe it moves outwards at the end of expiration
Abdominal wall moves outwards	Abdominal wall moves inwards.
Accessory muscles of respiration contract	
Nostrils dilate.	

Color becomes pale or cyanosed.
Pulse rate rises and later becomes irregular.
Blood pressure may rise at first but if obstruction is severe or prolonged the blood pressure falls.
Temperature may rise, especially in children where a combination of oxygen lack, carbon dioxide retention and the extra work involved in breathing often produce convulsions.
Patient becomes irrational, restless or unconscious or more deeply comatose.

lost its rigidity or tone, so that it falls back against the posterior pharyngeal wall. Immediate action is vital. The nurse restores the passage of air to and from the lungs by hooking the tongue forwards with her finger or with the aid of tongue forceps.

As soon as possible the patient is placed on his side, for two reasons: first to allow drainage from the mouth and nose of any vomit that may be present; and second, to allow the tongue, due to its own weight, to fall forward away from the pharyngeal wall thus helping to restore normal ventilation.

Following either or both of the above procedures, the next step is to maintain the patency of the airway by supporting the chin and by insertion of an oral airway.

SUPPORTING THE CHIN
Methods
Various techniques of supporting the chin are described. Consequently,

different instructions from different tutors can confuse the student nurse. Basically it matters not which method she adopts so long as it permits unobstructed respiration.

The maneuver depends on the tongue's attachment to the mandible. Elevation of the chin drags the tongue away from the posterior pharyngeal wall. The chin is raised to a position usually adopted when one sniffs suspiciously on becoming aware of an unexpected or unfamiliar aroma.

Another method is to elevate the chin and simultaneously pull the jaw forward. This maneuver depends on the mandible being L shaped. Standing at the head of the patient, the nurse places a hand on each side of the patient's face (Figure 17.1). Her little and ring fingers pull forward the upright portions (rami) of the mandible. Her middle and index fingers lift up the horizontal part (body) of the mandible. The thumbs rest on the cheek.

Precautions
The above maneuvers do not always guarantee unimpeded ventilation. The nurse must simultaneously listen to the patient's intake and output of air. To do this she must bend over the patient frequently so that her ear is within a few centimetres of the airway. She can then alter the position of the patient's head or adjust her support to his chin until she finds the position where the patient's respiratory exchange is best.

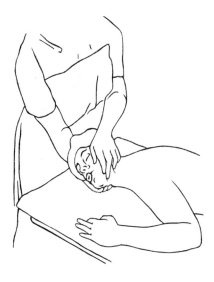

Figure 17.1   Supporting the chin

Dangers

Air can enter either the nose or mouth. Nasal entry is prevented by secretions, a swollen nasal mucous membrane, polyps, a deflected nasal septum, a broken nose or the presence of nasal packs inserted after nose operations. In these circumstances approximation of the lips completes the obstruction. Such conditions always demand the insertion of an oral airway. If, however, an airway is not instantly available the nurse must elevate the chin with one hand and separate the lips with a finger and thumb of the other hand.

Care is necessary in the edentulous patient especially in the old and the very young. Loss of dental support leaves the lips as a floppy fleshy mass that can, on chin elevation, bunch up and block the nostrils. Here again the nurse separates the lips with the fingers or preferably with the help of an oral airway.

ORAL AIRWAYS

The main function of the oral airway is to help to prevent respiratory obstruction. It separates the lips and teeth and prevents the tongue from coming into contact with the posterior pharyngeal wall. It facilitates the aspiration of pharyngeal secretions, prevents the awakening patient biting the endotracheal tube and provides a space in which to insert a mouth gag if the patient subsequently vomits solid material which needs removal by fingers or forceps.

Size of airway

Airways are graded in size starting with the smallest 00 and then getting progressively larger from size 0 to 4.

Babies up to 1 year old require size 00 or 0
Children from 1–5 years old require size 0 or 1
Children from 5 years old up to adult age require size 1 or 2
Adults require size 2, 3 or 4.

Correct choice of airway is important. Too small a size fails to bypass the relaxed tongue. If too large it irritates the pharynx causing the patient to retch or vomit unless he is deeply unconscious.

Precautions in airway insertion (Illustrated in Figures 17.2–17.11)
(1) The metal flange

When in correct position the proximal end of the airway rests between the bite of the front teeth, with the flange just in front of the lips. From the flange backwards, for 1.25 cm (½ inch) the rubber or plastic is lined by a protective sleeve of metal which prevents the airway being bitten and occluded. If the airway is left protruding from the mouth and the patient bites distal to the metal sleeve, or if the metal sleeve is missing,

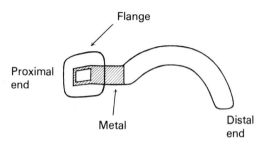

Figure 17.2   Oral airway

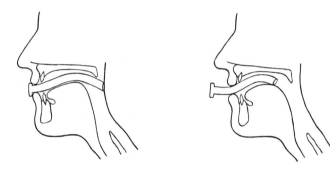

Figure 17.3 Airway in contact with the pharynx – can produce vomiting on recovery from anesthesia

Figure 17.4 Airway pulled away from the pharyngeal wall which is therefore not stimulated

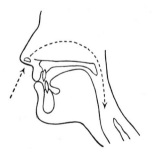   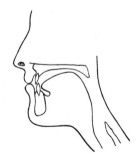

Figure 17.5 Lips together, air can enter through nose

Figure 17.6 Lips together, nose obstructed. Air cannot enter through lips or nose. Remedy – separate lips, insert airway – air can enter larynx

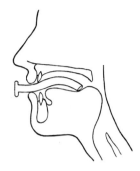

Figure 17.7 Too small an airway pushes tongue against the pharyngeal wall

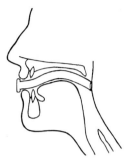

Figure 17.8 Too large an airway. Blockage due to pressing against the pharyngeal wall

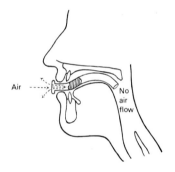

Figure 17.9 Blocked airway

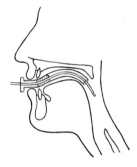

Figure 17.10 Catheter inserted allows air to pass. Obstruction relieved

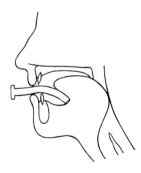

Figure 17.11 Airway inserted under tongue – complete obstruction

the lumen may be reduced or even cease to exist. Both effects cause differing degrees of respiratory obstruction especially if he is unable to breathe through his nose.

(2) *Relationship with tongue*
It may appear ridiculous to mention that the airway must be placed along the top of the tongue. Nevertheless, unless care is exercised it is easy to insert the airway underneath the tip of the tongue so that the tongue is forced upwards and backwards towards the roof of the mouth causing complete respiratory obstruction and the rapid onset of cyanosis. Such a mistake is most likely to occur in the small infant or a patient of any age with a dry mouth, often following the injection of atropine, when the tongue can literally stick to the palate. This is why some instructors advise the airway to be three-quarters inserted with the distal end first pointing upwards. Then the airway is rotated through 180° so that the distal end points downwards towards the larynx.

(3) *Protection of fraenum*
A further danger of introducing the airway beneath the tip of the tongue is the possible tearing of the fold of mucous membrane, the fraenum, which extends from the tongue to the floor of the mouth.

(4) *Care of lips*
Insertion of the airway is invariably followed by elevation of the chin. When the airway is advanced, the lips must not be rolled inwards and caught between the teeth and the airway. Biting the lips in this way can cause very unpleasant, painful and disfiguring ulceration which may take 7–10 days to heal.

Precautions after insertion
(1) *Confirm patency of airway*
Insertion of the airway does not guarantee that all is well. The nurse places her ear close to the patient's mouth and confirms there is a free flow of air through the airway. She also confirms that other signs of respiratory obstruction (p. 167) are absent. She may have to flex or extend the patient's head until she finds a suitable position which ensures a clear airway. Once established the ideal position is maintained because movement may then jeopardize the free air movements and also stimulate the posterior pharyngeal wall.

(2) *Avoid stimulation of posterior pharyngeal wall*
Slight stimulation of the posterior pharyngeal wall may make the patient swallow and hold his breath. More pronounced stimulation can cause retching and vomiting. If swallowing or breath holding do occur the nurse confirms that the jaw is elevated and then flexes or extends the head slightly. If swallowing continues or breathing does not return she

keeps the head in the same position with the chin raised, but withdraws the airway 1 cm out of the mouth. Should these maneuvers be ineffective the airway is removed. The patient is carefully observed. If, after a few seconds, spontaneous respiration returns but the lips or tongue are seen to obstruct respiration, then a smaller airway is inserted.

Duration of airway insertion
The airway is kept in the mouth until the nurse is sure that the patient is capable of sustaining an unobstructed airway. She is guided by several signs.

Signs of recovery
Recovery from a short anaesthetic in the Accident and Emergency department is usually rapid. The patient often spits out his airway. To do this he has to open his mouth and push the airway with his tongue. This requires restoration of power or muscle tone in the tongue. If this muscle tone is sufficient to push out an airway it is adequate to render the tongue powerful or stiff enough to prevent it falling backwards into the pharynx.

Gagging and retching
Some patients push or pull out their own airway and it is the routine of some teachers to instruct the nurse to leave the airway in position until this action is accomplished. Although this instruction is basically sound, some patients start to 'gag' on the airway and retch or vomit. In these circumstances the nurse is advised to withdraw the airway 1 cm away from the posterior pharyngeal wall. If the patient settles down again she is justified in waiting until he eventually discards the airway. On the other hand, if retching persists one teaching is to remove the airway. Removal at this stage may not be followed by the onset of vomiting but if it does occur the nurse may find the patient's mouth full of vomit and his teeth tightly clenched; she is unable to open the mouth and apply suction. Therefore, because of these possible eventualities, it is unwise to instantly remove the airway in a retching or vomiting patient. The other safer alternative, if the initial withdrawal of 1 cm leaves the patient still retching or vomiting is to withdraw the airway further so that only 2 cm of it remain in the mouth. The purpose of this maneuver is to keep the teeth separated. Even if the patient bites on the airway the small gap left between the teeth allows insertion of a mouth gag or sucker, thus allowing vomit to be removed.

Care after removal of the airway
Occasionally the patient ejects his airway, yet tends to become obstructed due to the absence of teeth and a blocked nose. Inspiratory

effort is accompanied by a sucking in of the cheeks and lips but with little or no entry of air through the mouth. This type of patient needs the assistance of the nurse in the separation of his lips or removal of mucus from the nostrils. Usually within a few minutes further recovery of consciousness is accompanied by the ability of the patient to open his mouth and breathe properly. With few exceptions, all unconscious patients should be placed in the lateral position (p. 180). The edentulous patient with floppy lips will benefit, even when almost fully conscious, because the lips will tend to hang open and thus allow unimpeded ventilation.

If separation of the lips does not restore unobstructed breathing the nurse hooks the tongue forward with her finger and reinserts the airway. Care is necessary in this maneuver if the patient has teeth. She should never insert her finger into such a patient's mouth unless she has the mouth opened by means of a mouth gag. Even a child of 3 years of age who clamps his teeth together can make the victim scream with pain. There is no need to elucidate on the damage that can be caused by the teeth of a fully grown adult.

NASOPHARYNGEAL AIRWAY

Inability to open the mouth because of spasm, swelling or damage may prevent insertion of an oral airway. Such obstruction inside the mouth is often effectively bypassed by means of a nasopharyngeal airway.

The nasopharyngeal airway is basically a short endotracheal tube (Figure 17.12). Its bore is similar but it is only about 13 cm (5 in) long and has a flange at its proximal end, which stops it slipping into the nose. An ordinary endotracheal tube serves the same purpose but in this case a safety pin is inserted through its proximal end to prevent its inhalation (Figure 17.13).

It is introduced into either nostril and passed backwards through the nasopharynx and into the oropharynx, thus separating the tongue from the posterior pharyngeal wall and helping to restore the airway.

Technique of introduction

The distal 4–5 cm (1½–2 in) is lubricated with jelly, or an analgesic cream. The nurse stands at the head of the patient and takes hold of the airway as if it were a dart. The tip, pointing forward, is inserted into the patient's nostril. At this stage it is important to remember that the nasal passages pass backwards, parallel to the roof of the mouth. Therefore, the airway is pushed in a backward and not an upward direction. Firm yet gentle pressure is necessary to direct the airway towards the pharynx. If any obstruction is encountered the nurse withdraws the airway 1 cm, rotates it through 45° and makes a further attempt to proceed. Failure demands a further rotation of 45°. Occasionally the

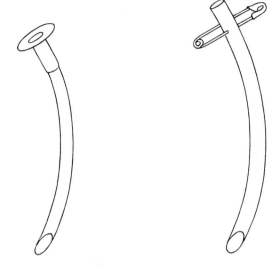

Figure 17.12 Naso-pharyngeal airway

Figure 17.13 Cut down endotracheal tube with safety pin

airway may have to be rotated almost around a full circle before it slips past the obstruction. Inability to pass the airway demands trial in the other nostril without trying too hard and too long on the first side which can damage the nasal mucous membrane.

In spite of gentleness, bleeding can occur and the patient is therefore maintained in the lateral position to prevent blood entering the larynx following successful or attempted introduction of the airway.

Inhalation of foreign material

Before discussing the prevention and relief of asphyxia caused by the inhalation of foreign material, it is necessary to understand the physiological mechanisms involved in breathing, swallowing and coughing.

Behind the nose and mouth is a space, the pharynx, the upper part being called the nasopharynx and the lower part the oropharynx. The stream of inspired air, entering through the nose, passes into and through the nasopharynx to enter the oropharynx. Air entering through the mouth moves immediately into the oropharynx.

Food, after being chewed, and drink at the start of the swallowing process, also enter the oropharynx.

The oropharynx is therefore a common cavity where the air and food streams meet. Then they separate, the air passing forwards through the

larynx and into the trachea, whereas the food and drink pass backwards
to enter the esophagus on their way to the stomach.

Figure 17.14 shows that the air stream and the food and drink stream
cross each other, just above the point where the pharynx divides into the
larynx and esophagus. Some mechanism is therefore essential to
separate these two streams in order to ensure that the air from the
oropharynx enters the lungs and that the food and drink enter only the
esophagus.

Separation of the two streams is accomplished by involuntary
muscular coordination but special protective anatomical and physiological mechanisms afford further security against accidental
inhalation of food or drink into the lower respiratory passages.

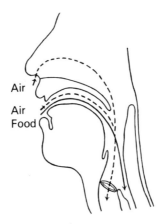

Figure 17.14   Air and food streams crossing in pharynx

PROTECTIVE MECHANISMS
Vocal cords
The entrance to the larynx is guarded by two muscular strands of tissue
covered by epithelium. Besides their role as protectors of the larynx
they also regulate the tone of the voice. Their anterior ends are always
close to each other but their posterior ends can move apart. Divergence
of the posterior ends is known as separation or abduction of the cords,
and this helps to produce a low note during speech. Convergence or
adduction of the cords raises the tone of the voice. This explains the
high pitched crowing sound that is produced when closure is almost
complete in the condition known as laryngeal spasm (p. 177). Complete
approximation of the cords to each other forms a total barrier to the
entry of food, drink, gastric contents and other foreign material.

Inhibition of respiration
Further protection of the bronchi is afforded by the temporary cessation of breathing whilst swallowing is taking place thus preventing food being sucked into the larynx.

Inhibition of swallowing
Temporary abolition of swallowing occurs when breathing is in progress. This prevents food reaching the esophagus during respiration or entering the larynx.

The nurse who is willing to spend a few seconds on paying attention to her own breathing and swallowing will soon learn that she cannot swallow and breathe at the same time.

Although the above mechanisms are usually extremely efficient, mistakes can occur in both the conscious and the unconscious patient.

In the conscious patient, food and drink occasionally go 'down the wrong way' and come into contact with the vocal cords. Immediately they clamp together to close off the larynx so that unwanted material cannot get into the bronchial tree. Closure is so complete that air too is unable to pass between them. Normal breathing does not resume until the foreign material is removed by the cough reflex. This reflex provokes an immediate reaction, that is an instant desire to cough. Coughing requires a forceful expulsion of air from the chest, usually provided by the expiratory reserve volume (p. 146) which may suffice to produce a few small coughs and thereby eject the offending material. If, however, irritation of the vocal cords persists then further coughing is provoked but, in order to cough air out of the chest, air must first be allowed into the lungs. This leaves the vocal cords in a dilemma with the choice of keeping any lurking foreign material out of the chest and at the same time causing their owner to suffocate, or to allow air to enter the lungs with a possibility of inhaling undesirable material. Naturally the cords do the latter but they are very cautious to the extent they open. At first their separation is slight and a small volume of air is inspired through the slit. This causes the high pitched crowing sound of laryngeal spasm. The condition is appropriately named because it is due to persistent contraction of the muscles within the vocal cords. Entry of sufficient air into the lungs initiates the coughing mechanism, the chest wall contracts, pressure builds up in the lungs and suddenly the vocal cords open. Any foreign material overlying the cords is blown towards the mouth. The vocal cords again go into spasm and the whole process is repeated. Coughing becomes more and more powerful, and the spasm less and less marked as the irritation decreases in severity. When irritation is no longer present, the cords return to their normal activity and regular respiration is restored.

In the unconscious patient, unconsciousness may be accidental due to injury or disease or it may be intentional during the induction, maintenance of, and recovery from anesthesia. Irrespective of the cause, vomit, blood, pus or excessive saliva may exist in the mouth or pharynx, all potentially lethal in that their inhalation can cause laryngeal spasm and atelectasis. These dangers are imminent because of the inability to cough. Loss of the cough reflex in coma and anesthesia is due to depression of the central control mechanism of the brain, loss of sensation in the vocal cords and their inability to contract effectively: they are asleep like the rest of the body. Any blood, perhaps from a lacerated tongue, or vomit which strays onto the vocal cords is ignored and runs or is sucked into the lungs. Because spasm is absent there may be no warning of the events taking place until the patient becomes cyanosed and maybe dies.

In the semi-conscious patient partial recovery from anesthesia or drowsiness, following head injury or overdosage of drugs, presents a response which is a mixture of that shown by the fully conscious and the unconscious patient.

At this stage the vocal cords have regained their protective rôle but the cough reflex remains partially ineffective. The irritation caused by the foreign material causes them to approximate. They later relax a little to allow a limited volume of air to enter the lungs, but the attempted cough is too weak to dislodge and eject the foreign material. Laryngeal spasm continues and the lack of oxygen causes a progressively deeper degree of cyanosis.

The nurse must know how to deal with these problems and, what is even more important, how to prevent their occurrence.

Regurgitation and vomiting

In the conscious patient the chewing and swallowing of food usually results in the swallowing of air, the amount of which varies with personal habits. Gas production in the stomach depends upon the type of food ingested and upon its reaction with the gastric juice. It is excessive in volume and offensive in odour if gastric emptying is delayed in conditions such as pyloric stenosis. Most swallowed air or gas is returned quietly to the mouth. Occasionally, however, it is accompanied by a little gastric juice or partially digested food whose silent appearance, without conscious effort, often startles the person concerned. This process is known as regurgitation.

Vomiting is the other means by which the stomach empties its contents but entails considerable muscular effort, especially by the abdominal muscles.

During regurgitation and vomiting respiration stops, the cords come together and close the larynx. At an opportune moment any gastric contents in the mouth and pharynx are spat out or reswallowed.

In the unconscious (comatose or anesthetized) patient regurgitation and vomiting also occur. Regurgitation is particularly dangerous because it occurs silently, without effort on the part of the patient.

Vomiting too is dangerous but often the nurse is warned by the patient retching or by the contraction of his abdominal muscles. On recovery from an anesthetic the patient often swallows and within the next 2 minutes he starts to vomit. The appearance of swallowing should always put the nurse on her guard.

Regurgitation and vomiting are dangerous in the unconscious patient because he is deprived of his protective reflexes. Entry of solid vomit into the larynx or bronchi can cause instant asphyxia and death. Liquid vomit flowing into the bronchial tree causes the collapse of lung tissue (atelectasis), irritation and perhaps severe bronchospasm. If the volume of inhaled gastric juice is considerable it has the same effect on the patient as putting his head in a bucket of water, in that he drowns in his own vomit.

Regurgitation and vomiting can occur at any time in the unconscious or semi-conscious patient especially when recovering from an anaesthetic. Therefore, it is obvious that every precaution must be taken to protect the patient against the inhalation of his gastric contents.

PREVENTION OF INHALATION OF SWALLOWED MATERIAL
Two basic principles should be followed. First, prevent the foreign material from reaching the larynx. Second, if it does reach the larynx remove it as quickly as possible. These are accomplished by suitable posture, oral, nasal and pharyngeal toilet and sometimes by endotracheal intubation.

Posture
Because of the effect of gravity, fluid flows downhill. Therefore, the head should be maintained at a lower level than the larynx and trachea. Blood and vomit then flow away from the lungs into the pharynx and out of the mouth, or into the nasopharynx and nasal cavities and out of the nose.

Consequently, the nurse should avoid raising the head of a weak or unconscious vomiting or regurgitating patient above the horizontal, even when trying to catch the gastric contents in a receiver, otherwise some may enter the lungs. However, the head-down position is not completely satisfactory, if the patient lies on his back (supine), because half a cupful of vomit can be 'stored' in the nasopharynx of an unconscious patient. If his head is then elevated, or he starts to awaken and sit up, this 'stored' vomit pours into the larynx with the obvious consequences. Because of this possibility the unconscious patient should be placed not only head down but also on his side. Vomit then flows away from the lungs and out of the mouth and nose. It cannot pool in the nasopharynx if he lies on his side. Lying on the side is known as the lateral position and is described below.

The lateral position is maintained until the patient is sufficiently conscious to be able to cough effectively, talk coherently or forcibly grasp the nurse's hand.

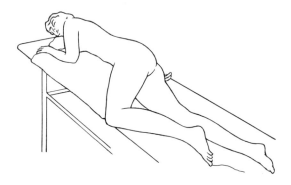

Figure 17.15   Right lateral position

The lateral position is the safest in the unconscious or recovering patient for the protection of the airway (Figure 17.15).

Most people go to sleep on their side, and if next time the nurse goes to bed, she adopts her natural lateral sleeping position she will discover she has placed her shoulders, hips, arms and legs in such a way, as described below, to ensure stability which is conducive to a good night's rest. She will then know how to posture her unconscious patient.

In the lateral position the upper shoulder rests a little in front of the lower shoulder. The upper arm is bent at the elbow so that the hand rests just below the chin. The lower arm too is bent at the elbow but to a lesser extent so that the hand rests on or beside the abdomen. An alternative position for the lower arm is to extend it and pull it backwards beneath the patient so that the hand rests behind the lower buttock.

The lower part of the body is stabilized by placing the hips in line with the shoulders, by having the lower leg straight and the upper leg bent at a right angle at the knee and to a lesser extent at the hip. Regarding the legs the order is 'top leg bent, bottom leg straight'.

Securing stability is very important, especially if the patient is heavier than the nurse, for if he falls over onto his face there is the danger of asphyxiation, his airway being obstructed by the coverings of the trolley (gurney). If he falls backwards he is less able to deal with any vomiting or regurgitation. Therefore, additional stability is assured by placing pillows in front of and behind the patient but not near his face.

If a tilting trolley or tilting bed is unavailable, one or two pillows are placed beneath the lower part of the chest, so that the mouth and pharynx reside at a lower level than the larynx. Positioning the pillows too high towards the head increases the chances of foreign material flowing into the lungs.

Minor alterations in posture are needed after some operations, especially after orthopedic procedures when the position is dictated by the plaster cast. Adequate padding, e.g. a pillow, is inserted between the plaster cast and any other part of the body with which it is in contact. This prevents crease formation on the inside of the plaster with its inherent dangers (p. 68), and avoids formation of a pressure sore or nerve palsy in the sound limb.

The lateral position in babies is as important as in the adult. Seeing a baby recovering from an anesthetic usually arouses sympathy and the desire to pick him up and give him a cuddle, especially if he is whimpering or sobbing. Because the protective reflexes have insufficiently recovered, lifting such a baby and cradling it in one's arms with the head elevated may sign its death warrant should it regurgitate and inhale gastric contents. The very ill, comatose or anesthetized baby must be given the 'full adult treatment'. He should be positioned head down, on his side, on an adult sized trolley, until the protective reflexes are fully alert. If circumstances prevail where the baby needs accommodating in a carrycot or incubator the same principles apply. The carrycot must be positioned or carried or the incubator tray tilted so that the baby's head is lower than its chest.

ENDOTRACHEAL INTUBATION
The presence of a cuffed endotracheal tube prevents vomit or other unwanted material from entering the lungs of the unconscious patient. The mechanism involved is discussed in Chapter 18.

18

Endotracheal intubation

F. WILSON

Endotracheal intubation usually lies within the province of the doctor, but there is no reason why the Accident and Emergency nurse should not become proficient in the art of intubation. In fact, it is desirable, and she should take every possible opportunity of watching how intubation is performed and be given practical training in the technique under the anesthetist's supervision. However, whether or not the nurse actually performs the intubation, it is essential for her to be acquainted with the purpose of the procedure, the type and size of equipment needed and its later management. Immediate intubation can be life-saving, but its speedy accomplishment and success often depends on the assistance of the nurse and her foresight in having the appropriate resuscitation equipment readily available.

The larynx
SIZE

The entrance to the larynx is guarded by the vocal cords which normally come together and move apart like 2 fans. The extent of the gap between the cords varies according to whether the owner decides to speak, swallow, cough or vomit. When they are fully apart the entrance to the adult larynx presents as a $\triangle$ shaped hole measuring 1.5 cm by 1.25 cm ($^5/_8''$ × $^1/_2''$). In the newborn baby the laryngeal entrance is 2.5 mm by 2 mm, which is only slightly wider than the thickness of a matchstick.

LARYNGEAL SWELLING

Swelling of the tissues at the entrance of the larynx is always dangerous, because any edema arising therein, due to roughness in endotracheal intubation, infection or growth, impinges on the airway and restricts the free passage of air to and from the lungs. The narrow bore of an infant's larynx demands special care during intubation because even slight swelling can reduce the lumen considerably, and cause severe respiratory obstruction.

A further precaution essential in avoiding laryngeal swelling is to choose an endotracheal tube whose size allows it to fit between but not press unduly against the vocal cords. The diameter is printed on the outside of the endotracheal tube and refers to its internal diameter. Appropriate sizes of tubes according to the patient's age are recorded in Table 18.1.

Table 18.1   Size of uncuffed oral endotracheal tubes for different age groups

Age	*Internal diameter*
Neonates (birth to 28 days)	
up to 2.0 kg (4.4 lb)	2.5 mm
Between 2.0 and 2.5 kg (4.4 and 5.5 lb)	3.0 mm
Between 2.5 and 3.5 kg (5.5 and 7.7 lb)	3.5 mm
Between 3.5 and 4.5 kg (7.7 and 9.9 lb)	4.0 mm
Infants	
Between 1 month and 1 year	4.0 mm
Between 1 year and 2 years	4.5 mm
Children	
Between 2 and 3 years	5.0 mm
Between 3 and 4 years	5.0 mm or 5.5 mm
Between 4 and 5 years	5.5 mm
Between 5 and 6 years	5.5 mm or 6.0 mm
Between 6 and 7 years	6.0 mm
Between 7 and 8 years	6.0 mm or 6.5 mm
Between 8 and 10 years	6.5 mm
Between 10 and 12 years	6.5 mm or 7.0 mm
Between 12 and 14 years	7.0 mm
Between 14 and 16 years	7.0 mm or 7.5 mm
Between 16 and 18 years	8.0 mm
Above 18 (female)	8.0 mm, 8.5 mm or 9 mm
Above 18 (male)	8.5 mm, 9 mm or 9.5 mm

Resistance in endotracheal tube

In order to avoid pressure on the vocal cords, the immediate response may perhaps be to select an endotracheal tube whose bore is too small. But, just as it is dangerous to select one too wide, it is also dangerous to choose one that is too narrow. To appreciate why this is so is demonstrated easily if the nurse carries out the following experiments upon herself.

She takes four endotracheal tubes whose sizes are 5.0 mm, 6.0 mm, 7.0 mm and 8.0 mm. If these are unavailable the same experiments can be performed by using endotracheal connectors (Figure 23.4), sizes 1, 2, 3 and 4, all of which should be available in Emergency and Anesthetic departments.

Experiment 1
She places one end of the 8.0 mm endotracheal tube (or size 4 endotracheal connector) in her mouth, purses her lips around it closely to ensure an airtight fit, and occludes her nostrils between finger and thumb, so that she cannot breathe through her nose. Air can then only enter her lungs via the endotracheal tube.

She breathes normally and notes how long she can breathe through the tube without distress. She will find breathing easy for as long as she wishes because the 8.0 mm bore is adequate to allow a sufficient tidal volume (p. 142) to pass through and ventilate her lungs. She can even breathe quickly and deeply without distress.

Experiment 2
Experiment 1 is repeated but with a size 7.0 mm tube (or size 3 endotracheal connector). The free entry and exit of air is again obvious but the rush of air is more pronounced. However, if she breathes deeply and quickly she finds that the supply of air does not appear to be quite as plentiful as it was during quiet respiration. Also she discovers that her respiratory muscles have to work harder than in experiment 1.

Experiment 3
Quiet breathing through a 6.0 mm tube (or size 2 endotracheal connector) is unpleasant after a few minutes and it soon becomes obvious that enough air cannot pass through the small bore to supply her needs. The inadequate bore has produced a degree of respiratory obstruction. After 2 or 3 minutes the feeling of suffocation forces her to abandon the experiment and rapidly take in a few gulps of air.

Experiment 4
Respiration through a 5.0 mm tube (or size 1 endotracheal connector) is possible for only 20–30 seconds. Almost at once she finds that both inspiration and expiration are prolonged in the attempt to obtain sufficient oxygen and to eliminate her carbon dioxide. The extra effort involved is seen by the increased muscular efforts of her chest and abdomen. At this stage she is experiencing the onset of asphyxia. Removal of the tube or connector from her mouth is followed by rapid deep breathing which continues until the oxygen and carbon dioxide in the alveolar air have returned to their normal levels.

INFORMATION GAINED FROM THE EXPERIMENTS

(1) On concluding these experiments the nurse should remember that they were performed on a conscious person, namely herself. She can stop the experiment whenever she wants. An unconscious patient cannot complain when the airway is inadequate. Such a patient with severe respiratory obstruction as exists in experiments 3 and 4 deteriorates rapidly as asphyxia becomes more prolonged and pronounced. If unrelieved the obstruction can cause death within a few minutes.

(2) The endotracheal tube must have as large a bore as possible to allow adequate ventilation yet not be so wide that it may damage the larynx.

(3) The bore of the endotracheal tube and the bore of the endotracheal connector both influence the quantity of air passing to and from the lungs. Therefore, it is essential to insert an endotracheal connector with a bore as wide as possible into the endotracheal tube, otherwise, although the bore of the endotracheal tube may be adequate, that of the endotracheal connector may be insufficient to achieve proper lung ventilation.

   Therefore, always insert the largest endotracheal connector which will fit into the appropriate endotracheal tube. To do this it is necessary to lubricate the connector with water, spirit or a spot of jelly.

(4) In the last two experiments the narrowness of the tube or connector interfered with the free flow of air, i.e., there was a noticeable increase in resistance to the passage of air. Such an increased resistance to breathing occurs in asthma where the narrowing of the bronchi due to spasm has the same effect as breathing through a 6.0 mm tube or size 2 endotracheal connector.

   Narrowing of the air passages occurs in bronchitis and emphysema because of the presence of secretions and the floppiness of the bronchioles arising from a loss of elastic tissue. Hence these conditions are included under the term 'obstructive airway disease' (p. 266). Another terminology says the patient suffers from airflow obstruction.

   Whenever the narrowing becomes severe the patient becomes distressed due to dyspnea (p. 265) and eventually he may pass into respiratory failure (p. 266)

(5) Because insertion of an endotracheal tube or endotracheal connector can themselves produce respiratory obstruction the nurse should record their size. If the patient shows signs later of

respiratory obstruction she is instantly able to assert, because the correct tube and connector were used, that some other factor must be the cause.

Length of endotracheal tube

Endotracheal tubes are made of rubber or plastic. They are plain, cuffed or armoured. They are classified further into oral and nasal types according to whether they are principally intended for introduction through the mouth or nose.

Choice of the correct length is very important. If it is too short it either does not reach or else it slips out of the larynx. If too long it slides into the right bronchus.

HOW TO CHOOSE THE LENGTH

All endotracheal tubes produced by the manufacturers are too long and a segment has to be cut from the proximal end which houses the endotracheal connector. The length of the endotracheal tube and therefore of the piece removed depends on whether the tube is passed orally or nasally and also on the patient's size and individual facial characteristics.

The proximal end should just protrude, by 0.5–1 cm, in front of the teeth or gums, or to a similar distance out of the nose. If it extends further outwards it is likely to be bitten or kink and the patient may asphyxiate.

The distal end, in an adult, should extend 5 cm (2 in) beyond the vocal cords otherwise any head movement may draw the endotracheal tube out of the larynx. If such a mishap is unnoticed, and the patient is being artificially ventilated, no air can enter the lungs and he will die. If having slipped out of the larynx, it slides backward into the esophagus the ventilator will blow up his stomach. Death may result from asphyxia or stomach rupture.

Too long a tube passes down the trachea and into the right bronchus. All the ventilation is restricted to the right bronchus and right lung, and the left bronchus and lung receive no ventilation at all. As a result the deoxygenated blood reaching the left lung leaves it as deoxygenated as when it arrives. This may cause cyanosis (p. 162), and the patient is said to have a 'shunt' (p. 239) because blood is shunted past lung tissue which is not ventilated. An endotracheal tube in a bronchus, be it left or right, causes a profound (manmade) shunt. Shunts also occur in disease when air is prevented from reaching the alveoli so that blood passes close by but is not oxygenated.

A pronounced shunt as occurs on intubation of the bronchus produces various degrees of asphyxia. The strong patient may survive for hours showing signs of sweating, tachycardia and increased carbon dioxide and lowered oxygen concentrations in his blood. The ill patient may be unable to stand even a slight degree of asphyxia and may soon perish.

Diagnosis of intubation of the bronchus is usually easy, but not always. The nurse or doctor listens to the chest with the aid of a stethoscope. Air entry just below the clavicles should sound equal on both sides. If air entry is not easily audible on the left the doctor should be informed. He will then withdraw the tube by 1–2 cm and listen again. An improvement in air entry into the left lung confirms that the tube is too long.

Another means of diagnosis is to take a chest X-ray which shows the position of the endotracheal tube and its relationship to the bronchi. Many endotracheal tubes incorporate a radio-opaque marker which helps in X-ray diagnosis but care must be taken not to confuse it with ECG leads or central venous pressure (CVP) lines (p. 138).

Advantages of endotracheal intubation

Endotracheal intubation relieves respiratory embarrassment in one or all of the following ways:

(1) It relieves obstruction in the mouth, oropharynx, and larynx (p. 166).
(2) It reduces dead space (p. 188).
(3) It allows aspiration of secretions from trachea and bronchi (p. 190).
(4) It provides a means through which mechanical ventilation of the lungs can be performed without having to contend with the movements of the vocal cords.
(5) It prevents the inhalation of vomit into the lungs (p. 179).

RELIEF OF OBSTRUCTION IN MOUTH, OROPHARYNX AND LARYNX
Respiratory obstruction in the mouth, oropharynx and larynx occurs as a result of trauma, infection, growths, burns or allergy. Endotracheal intubation bypasses the obstruction and restores the airway.

Although it is advisable to select an endotracheal tube whose size is appropriate to the age of the patient (Table 18.1), there are occasions where the lesion narrows the normal airway sufficiently to allow only the use of a tube with a much smaller bore. For example, a wasp sting or a growth near the larynx may permit the entry of only a 6 mm endotracheal tube whose length is usually suitable for a 10–12 year old. Such a tube would be too short in the adult and fail to reach the larynx. This is the only occasion where it is wise to use a new long *uncut* endotracheal tube as supplied by the manufacturer (p. 186).

Although the experiments on page 184 show that such a choice may appear unwise, because of the resistance to respiration, the intro- duction of a narrow endotracheal tube can be life-saving and keep the patient alive until a tracheostomy is performed.

If a suitable uncut endotracheal tube is unavailable, insertion of a plastic catheter through the larynx is perfectly suitable as a temporary measure.

If the above measures fail the resuscitator is left with the choice of getting below the obstruction by means of a rapid tracheostomy or by the insertion of one or two plastic cannulae, normally used for blood transfusion, through the crico-thyroid membrane. As the name suggests this membrane joins together the cricoid and thyroid cartilages.

REDUCTION OF DEAD SPACE
Reduction of the dead space (p. 151) allows a higher proportion of the tidal volume (p. 142) to enter the lungs so that endotracheal intubation is said to increase the effective tidal volume (p. 151).

Insertion of an endotracheal tube allows air to enter the trachea without having to pass through the mouth, nose, pharynx and larynx. Therefore, endotracheal intubation reduces the dead space so that it then consists of the internal volume of the endotracheal tube, the lower part of the trachea, the bronchi and the bronchioles. Tables 18.2–18.5 show the effect of endotracheal intubation on dead space and effective tidal volume.

	Table 18.2	Table 18.3	Table 18.4	Table 18.5
Tidal volume (ml)	350	275	275	300
Dead space (ml)	150	150	75	75
Effective tidal volume (ml)	200	125	200	225
	Before intubation	Before intubation	After intubation the dead space is halved	After intubation the dead space is halved

Tables 18.2 and 18.3 show that if the tidal volume is reduced from 350 ml to 275 ml, the effective tidal volume falls from 200 ml to 125 ml. But, Table 18.4 shows that reducing the dead space by endotracheal intubation restores the effective ventilation from 125 ml to 200 ml (Table 18.2). Therefore, the intubated patient with a tidal volume of 275 ml can ventilate his lungs as well as he could prior to intubation when his tidal volume was 350 ml.

Perusal of Tables 18.2 and 18.5 reveals that an intubated patient with a tidal volume of 300 ml can ventilate his lungs more effectively than a person whose tidal volume is 350 ml but who is not intubated. Unfortunately, he has to pay a penalty for this increased ventilation. Temporarily, he loses his voice and his ability to cough effectively, and he is deprived of the mechanisms that moisten the air which enters the lungs.

To take a further example, Figure 18.1 shows the tidal volumes achieved by two adult patients, A and B. While A has fairly adequate effective tidal volume, B can only maintain the same effective tidal volume if he is intubated.

Improvement in ventilation of the lungs by endotracheal intubation illustrates that it can be a life-saving procedure whenever there is

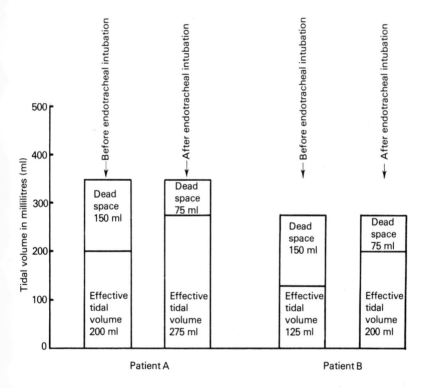

Figure 18.1 Diagram to illustrate in two patients, A & B:
    (1)   Endotracheal intubation reduces anatomical dead space to half
    (2)   Endotracheal intubation increases effective tidal volume

depression of the respiratory centre. Accidental or intentional over-dosage of drugs, or a head injury, may cause profound respiratory depression so that effective ventilation falls below that necessary to sustain life. Endotracheal intubation, besides securing the airway and bypassing the relaxed tongue may sufficiently improve ventilation to support the patient until the drug has been excreted, or the appropriate antidote has been given, or until he has recovered from his head injury.

If adequate ventilation is not re-established intermittent positive pressure ventilation (IPPV, p. 227) is started without delay and a decision is made whether to perform a tracheostomy. At this point it is useful to appreciate that some tracheostomies are performed with the aim of reducing the dead space. However, this problem is usually encountered in the intensive care unit. But, if the nurse follows the reasoning behind the statement 'endotracheal intubation reduces the dead space' she will have no difficulty in realizing that a tracheostomy tube does the same. A tracheostomy tube has one advantage in that it does not harm the vocal cords because it is inserted below the larynx.

Endotracheal suction
Suction can be applied by means of a catheter to the trachea and bronchi. It is performed when the patient is unable to cough up his own secretions. Such circumstances occur in the debilitated person, usually at one or other of the extremes of life, especially when mucus production is excessive as occurs in bronchitis and bronchopneumonia. Muscular incoordination or paralysis due to a stroke, poliomyelitis or the Guillain–Barré syndrome may prevent him from coughing effectively. Sputum accumulation can also follow a head injury, drug over-dosage or any type of coma.

Vomit, inhaled during coma or anesthesia, water following drowning, and blood aspirated into the bronchi after injury to the mouth, nose or throat are often removed successfully by suction catheter.

AIM OF SUCTION
The aim of suction is to improve the patency of the airway and restore adequate ventilation of the lungs.

A sudden abundance of foreign material in the trachea and bronchi is most likely to have unpleasant results causing death from asphyxia or coma due to 'respiratory failure' (p. 266). Lesser degrees of obstruction cause varying degrees of atelectasis and the possible development of bronchopneumonia.

TECHNIQUE OF SUCTION
The catheter should be sterile.

Before handling the catheter the nurse washes her hands, and preferably puts a disposable glove on the hand she intends to restrict to the handling of the catheter. The ungloved hand is used for unclean activities such as connecting the suction apparatus to the suction catheter.

Size of catheter
The correct size of the chosen catheter should be sufficient to allow the free passage of thick mucus, but should not exceed half the internal diameter of the endotracheal tube.

The catheter tip is first pushed into the collection of sputum, vomit or blood. After a brief period of suction, usually 2 or 3 seconds, the sputum enters the catheter and suction tubing. From this time on, continued suction serves no useful purpose and merely withdraws air from that part of the bronchial tree which contains the tip of the catheter. However, provided there is plenty of space between the outside of the catheter and the inside of the endotracheal tube, any air removed by the catheter tip is replaced immediately and freely by air from the outside atmosphere rushing downwards between catheter and tube. In these circumstances no harm comes to the patient so long as the period of suction is not unduly prolonged.

Incorrect size of catheter can lead to very serious consequences. If the catheter diameter is almost similar to that of the endotracheal tube and if suction is continued, after all the mucus has been removed, there is insufficient space between the catheter and tube for the inrush of air required to replace that being sucked up by the catheter. As a result, the suction apparatus draws air out of the lungs quicker than it is replaced, thus causing partial or complete pulmonary collapse and profound hypoxia. Possibly the patient may end up with a far more extensive atelectasis than if the sputum were allowed to remain.

Shape of catheter
Some designs of catheter have the tip angulated. By pointing the tip to the left or right, as the catheter is inserted, it is often possible to steer it into either of the main bronchi. On the other hand, advancement of a straight tipped catheter usually results in it entering the right main bronchus; the right bronchus, unlike the left, is more in a straight line with the trachea.

Lubrication of catheter
The catheter is lubricated by placing its distal 5 cm (2 in) in sterile normal saline, after which it is allowed to drain vertically for a few

seconds. Alternatively, a small amount of lubricating jelly applied with the gloved hand is equally effective.

Introduction of catheter

To avoid producing atelectasis due to prolonged suction it is advisable to apply the suction only during the time the catheter is being withdrawn. To achieve this aim various techniques are popular, all of which are satisfactory.

For example, the plain catheter, not attached to the suction apparatus, is advanced gently and as far as it will go down the endotracheal tube. It is then connected to the suction apparatus and suction applied as it is withdrawn.

Another method using the plain catheter is to insert into it the stem of a glass or plastic 'Y' piece (Figure 18.3). The bore of the 'Y' piece

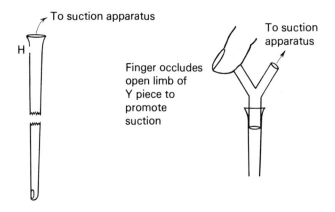

Figure 18.2 Straight catheter with hole (H) at proximal end

Figure 18.3 Y piece with catheter attached

should be as near as possible to the diameter of the catheter to enable air to pass freely through both its stem and 'limbs'. One limb of the 'Y' piece is joined to the suction apparatus. The second limb is left open to the atmosphere so that suction is ineffective until it is occluded by the nurse's finger.

An additional hole (H) is present in some types of catheter and is situated near its proximal end (Figure 18.2). Attachment of this type of catheter to the suction apparatus draws air up the catheter from the tip and also in through the hole. As with the 'Y' piece there is no danger of suction being applied to the lungs unless the hole (H) is occluded.

SUCTION IN THE APNEIC PATIENT

The patient may be unable to breathe spontaneously because of his injury or disease, or he may be rendered apnoeic by suxamethonium (succinylcholine, p. 219) or longer acting relaxants. Both types of patient require intermittent positive pressure ventilation (IPPV, p. 221) performed by bag and mask (p. 227) or by means of a ventilator (p. 223). In order to aspirate secretions from the bronchi, it is necessary to disconnect the endotracheal tube from the resuscitation apparatus. During this period of disconnection respiratory movements are at a standstill and the patient rapidly becomes hypoxic. Therefore, the nurse must be ready to insert the catheter into the endotracheal tube immediately it is disconnected. Reconnection after withdrawal of the catheter must be instantaneous in order to allow ventilation to restart. If further attempts at suction are needed, it is wise to alternate short periods of suction with IPPV, rather than trying to remove all the foreign material at once by sliding the catheter repeatedly up and down the trachea. The latter technique is most likely to cause hypoxia, asphyxia, atelectasis and heart failure. If reflex bradycardia develops during endobronchial suction then the suction must be discontinued immediately.

Choice of plain or cuffed endotracheal tube

The decision whether a plain or cuffed endotracheal tube is needed depends on the condition requiring endotracheal intubation. This decision can be made and the subsequent management changed if the doctor and nurse understand the movements of air that take place within and around the endotracheal tube.

ROUTES OF AIR FLOW USING THE PLAIN TUBE

Provided the vocal cords can separate from each other, air can pass from the atmosphere by two different routes. On inspiration air enters the endotracheal tube and passes into the trachea where it is joined by a smaller quantity of air which has entered by the normal route between the vocal cords. During expiration air flow is reversed, making its exit from the lungs using the same routes by which it entered. Because during respiration air can pass to and fro between the outer wall of the tube and the tracheal mucosa, it is obvious that secretions or vomit can run alongside the tube and enter the bronchi. Therefore, a plain tube can guarantee the airway in that it bypasses the relaxed tongue, but it is unable to completely prevent the aspiration of foreign material although its presence between the cords prevents the inhalation of the larger constituents of solid vomit. Full protection is provided only by the cuffed type of endotracheal tube.

The plain tube is unsuitable for IPPV because when air is pumped through it some of the air enters the lungs but much escapes upwards between the endotracheal tube and the trachea eventually escaping between the tube and the vocal cords. If this leakage is marked, such as occurs in the combination of a wide laryngeal aperture with a narrow bore tube, then it is impossible to inflate the lungs sufficiently well to produce an adequate tidal exchange.

ROUTES OF AIR FLOW WHEN USING THE CUFFED TUBE
Correct inflation (p. 195) of the cuff obliterates the space between the endotracheal tube and the tracheal wall, thereby dividing the trachea into an upper and a lower half. The upper part of the trachea is in communication with the larynx and the lower part is in communication with the bronchi and lungs.

During spontaneous ventilation the inflated cuff prevents the inspiration and expiration of air between the endotracheal tube and the tracheal wall. In IPPV any gas pumped down the endotracheal tube has no alternative but to enter the lungs; it cannot leak past the cuff to escape out through the larynx.

The cuffed endotracheal tube with its cuff deflated acts in an identical manner to the plain tube and either can be used in an emergency to relieve a mechanical obstruction.

THE CUFF AND PILOT BALLOON
Correct inflation of the cuff serves two useful functions when it obliterates the space between the endotracheal tube and the tracheal lining. First, the cuff prevents regurgitated gastric contents, saliva and nasal secretions from entering the lower part of the trachea, the bronchi and their smaller divisions within the lung. Second, the cuff ensures that air, oxygen and anesthetic gases, which may have to be pumped into the endotracheal tube, will enter the lungs and not escape through the larynx.

Inflation of the cuff is achieved by the introduction of air through a syringe into the pilot tubing. After inflation to the required size, the cuff is prevented from deflating by clamping the pilot tubing with a pair of artery forceps between the syringe and the pilot balloon (Figure 18.4), or by the insertion of an attached spigot. The pilot balloon informs the observer whether the cuff is inflated and that it is airtight. Leakage of air from the inflated cuff or from the pilot balloon or its tubing causes the balloon to deflate. This happens when either the cuff, balloon or tubing is punctured or perished. Deflation of the pilot balloon also occurs when the pair of artery forceps or the spigot is faulty or has been incorrectly applied.

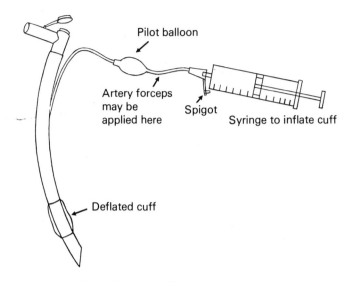

Pilot balloon

Artery forceps
may be
applied here

Spigot

Syringe to inflate cuff

Deflated cuff

Figure 18.4 A cuffed endotracheal tube

Testing the cuff and pilot balloon for leaks
It is essential to test the cuff before the endotracheal tube is inserted into
the trachea. The nurse attaches a 5 or 10 ml syringe to the pilot tubing.
She inserts 2 or 3 ml of air into the pilot tubing so that the cuff inflates.
She then applies a pair of artery forceps to the pilot tubing (or inserts
the spigot) and gently squeezes the balloon between finger and thumb
so that some of the air from the balloon is forced into the cuff itself.
Provided that the artery forceps are applied securely, and provided
neither cuff nor balloon is perforated, the balloon should return to its
original size and shape when it is no longer compressed. Testing the cuff
and balloon is especially important with those endotracheal tubes made
of rubber and which have been re-sterilized. Quantities of air greater
than 2–3 ml should not be introduced into the pilot tubing, otherwise
the cuff is stretched and weakened, and is more likely to rupture or
herniate inside the patient.

During testing, the cuff should inflate uniformly. Formation of a
bleb shows that a localized weakness exists. Such a tube should be
discarded.

Insufficient inflation of a cuff inside the trachea allows secretions to
trickle down past the cuff, so that collapse of part of the lung tissue may
arise if these secretions obstruct the bronchi or bronchioles. Also,
leakage of air or gas past the cuff renders IPPV less efficient.

Excessive inflation of a cuff inside the trachea serves no useful purpose, and may be dangerous because the excessive pressure which it exerts on the tracheal lining compresses the underlying blood vessels, and so deprives the tracheal mucosa of its oxygen supply. Necrosis of the mucosa can occur so that sloughing and infection arise where the cuff has pressed against the trachea. This is particularly likely to occur in the hypotensive patient. Eventually, destruction of tissue beneath the mucosa can weaken the cartilaginous tracheal rings so that they bulge outwards. Therefore, the amount of air injected into the cuff should be just sufficient to occlude the space between the cuff and the trachea. Obviously the diameter of the trachea varies from patient to patient so that more air is necessary within the cuff to prevent the aspiration of secretions in a patient with a wide trachea than is required when the trachea is of a narrower bore. Similarly, a narrow endotracheal tube requires more air in the cuff than when a wider tube is used. The exact amount of air required for inflation of the cuff can be decided if anaesthetic apparatus is available (see below), but if this is not to hand 3–5 ml of air are usually satisfactory in the adult patient.

When IPPV is performed, certain precautions must be taken. The expiratory valve is temporarily but completely closed and the reservoir bag squeezed. At the same time, air is introduced through a syringe into the cuff until the hiss of escaping gas between tracheal wall and cuff cannot be heard. The expiratory valve must not be kept closed for more than a few seconds (p. 230).

19

Apparatus for general anesthesia

A. KILPATRICK

The Boyle anesthetic machine

The Boyle anesthetic machine, first introduced in 1917, is basically a bank of flowmeters controlling the quantities of oxygen, nitrous oxide, carbon dioxide and, in some, cyclopropane, which are delivered to the patient; one or more vaporizers through which these gases may be passed; and some sort of tubing to deliver the gases to the patient.

(1) FLOWMETERS

These appear as vertical clear glass tubes along which a gas flows at a rate controlled by a rotating knob, and is measured by observing the level which a bobbin reaches as it is lifted by the flowing gas. The lightweight metallic bobbin is shaped like a short cylinder with a conical lower end, and is marked by spiral indentations which cause it to spin steadily as it rises in the flowing gas. The flow rate, in litres per minute (l/min), is measured by reading the marking on the flowmeter tube opposite the upper flat surface of the bobbin. In those machines which have round ball-like bobbins, the reading is taken opposite the centre of the balls. Each flowmeter is designed for a specific gas. It is usual for flowmeters for oxygen and for nitrous oxide to be capable of delivering 8 and 12 l/min respectively while those for carbon dioxide deliver up to 2 l/min with marks every 100 or 200 ml. Cyclopropane flowmeters are of narrower bore and give flowrates up to 1 or 2 l/min in increments of 50 ml. To turn on a gas flow the control knob is turned in an anti-clockwise direction and in the reverse direction, i.e. clockwise, to turn it off again. Turning off a flowmeter must be done gently so that the valve seating is not damaged.

(2) VAPORIZERS

If a volatile liquid anaesthetic agent such as diethyl ether or trichloroethylene is placed in a container and gas is allowed to flow over its surface, the gas leaves the container carrying some of the vapour given off by that liquid. The amount of vapour given off depends upon two main factors. First, the higher the temperature of the liquid the more easily is the liquid vaporized. Second, if the gas is bubbled through the liquid it has a more intimate contact with the liquid and so is able to carry away more vapour than a gas merely flowing over its surface.

Formerly, the only vaporizers available were simply glass bottles into which the selected volatile anesthetic was poured. A control lever at the upper end allowed a variable quantity of gas, usually a mixture of oxygen and nitrous oxide, to pass over or through the liquid. Such vaporizing chambers are still seen on modern anesthetic machines though they are seldom used. They do not supply a measured or constant vapour strength because the passage of gas over or through the liquid cools it and so reduces the amount of vapour given off. The anesthetist varies the amount of gas flowing over the liquid by using the lever and by manipulating a metal sleeve which directs the gases downwards onto or below the surface of the anesthetic agent. The sole criterion for varying the controls is clinical judgement acquired with experience.

However, it is more usual nowadays to use a specially constructed vaporizer for each anesthetic agent. These are graduated to denote the vapour strength delivered to the patient, and are constructed in such a way that they compensate for changes in liquid temperature and in gas flow. Vaporizers are in use which deliver halothane (Fluothane), enflurane (Ethrane) and trichloroethylene (Trilene) in known vapour strengths. Each vaporizer must only be used with the agent for which it is constructed. While the standard anesthetic machines in hospital departments usually carry the larger types of vaporizer there are often smaller and lighter vaporizers on portable anesthetic machines which also accurately deliver the vapour strength indicated on the control.

(3) GAS CYLINDERS

These are just containers whose function is to store gases, and enable them to be transferred from the site of manufacture to the place where the gases are to be administered. They are heavy, expensive, often cumbersome, are usually rented by the user from the manufacturer, and each one is designed for a specific gas. The gas for which each is made is indicated by the color of the cylinder. In the United Kingdom, nitrous oxide cylinders are blue, oxygen cylinders are black with white 'shoulders', carbon dioxide cylinders are grey and cyclopropane cylinders are small and orange in color. However, other countries adopt different colour schemes so any nurse working abroad must never rely on the colour code of her home country. She must always read the label displayed on the cylinder and find out the color code operative in her new environment. In addition, the cylinders are available in various standard sizes, some small to make them readily portable for domiciliary use, while others are tall and relatively heavy, for use in pipeline systems. Each cylinder has its empty weight plainly marked on it, and this is particularly useful because with some gases the only way to know the amount of gas contained within the cylinder is to weigh the cylinder and its contents. Strange as it may at first appear, a gas does have weight and this weight, while not appreciable while the gas is in its normal state, is significant when the gas is compressed in a cylinder. A fact, not readily obvious, is that gases contained within cylinders are not all in the same physical state. Oxygen for example, in a cylinder is present in gaseous form and a pressure gauge connected to the opened cylinder measures the pressure being exerted by the oxygen within the confines of the cylinder. When the cylinder is full the pressure is around 1950 lb per sq. inch (p.s.i.), equivalent to 133 times atmospheric pressure. As the oxygen flows out during its administration, the pressure falls in proportion to the gas which remains. The pressure is, therefore, around 975 p.s.i. (66 atmospheres) when the cylinder is only half full and so on.

However the situation is different with nitrous oxide, because this gas when compressed soon starts to liquify. As the compression occurs, more and more gas liquifies until eventually the 'full' cylinder, used on the anesthetic machine, contains 80% of its nitrous oxide as a liquid and the other 20% in gaseous form. A pressure gauge attached to an opened nitrous oxide cylinder, registers the pressure exerted by the gaseous nitrous oxide. When some of the gas is allowed to escape, the remaining gas temporarily exerts less pressure on the liquid nitrous oxide which takes the opportunity to become a gas again and takes up the space vacated by the gas previously released. This is a continuous process but the overall effect is that, as the nitrous oxide flows from the cylinder during use, the gauge measuring the gas pressure remains at the same level – around 750 p.s.i. (51 atmospheres) – until all the liquified nitrous oxide has been converted to a gaseous state. At this point, and not before, the registered pressure begins to fall. Once it does begin to fall, it falls quickly and quite soon the cylinder empties. This rapid fall in pressure occurs because there is no liquid nitrous oxide left to be converted to gaseous nitrous oxide to replace the released gas. Therefore, continued use at this stage causes a rapid fall in registered pressure. Every pressure gauge has a red warning area on its dial. Entry of the indicator into this area tells the anesthetist that it is time to bring a fresh cylinder into use, to turn off the near empty cylinder and replace it with a full one.

In the act of vaporizing from the liquid state, the nitrous oxide loses latent heat and the cylinder becomes very cold and usually 'frosts up' on its outer surface near its lower end. Nitrous oxide cylinders – and cylinders containing any other gas present in liquid and gaseous forms – must be used in the vertical position with the gas outlet end of the cylinder at a higher lever than the closed end. This is so that the gas vapour and not the liquid gas is at the exit from the cylinder.

Every anesthetic machine has pins which fit into matching holes on the cylinders near the gas outlet. The arrangement of pins and matching holes are different for every gas so that this pin index system makes it impossible to fit the wrong type of cylinder to an anesthetic machine. A typical layout is illustrated in Figure 19.1. Carbon dioxide is stored in its cylinder in a similar gaseous and liquid state. Its gaseous pressure is 735 p.s.i. (50 atmospheres). Cyclopropane is stored in cylinders as a gas and at a relatively low pressure, 75 p.s.i. (5.1 atmospheres), and because of this does not require the use of a reducing valve (p. 201).

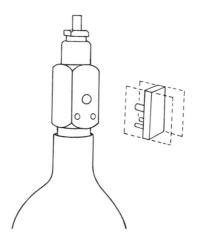

Figure 19.1   Pin index system

Treatment and handling of cylinders

As cylinders contain gases under considerable pressure it should be realised that they must be handled with great care. Each one is opened by turning a removable key which releases the gas from the opening. Before fitting a cylinder to an anesthetic machine the key should be turned gently and very carefully to allow a small escape of gas. This is done to blow out any dust which may have gathered around the opening. While this is being done, care is taken to see that neither fingers nor face are near the opening, lest the rapid escape of the gas causes friction burns of the skin or blows dust into the eyes which can further be damaged by the blast of gas. Grease must never be applied to cylinders, particularly those containing oxygen.

REDUCING VALVES AND PIPELINES
Each cylinder is fitted with a reducing valve, which reduces the high pressure of the gas within the cylinder to a lower, more manageable level and which can be accurately controlled by the flowmeters. The reduction of pressure also prevents the patient's lungs being exposed to high cylinder pressures, which would undoubtedly cause them damage.

However, while it is worthwhile for nurses to appreciate the significance of pressure gauges and reducing valves on cylinders, many work in hospitals where the nitrous oxide and oxygen are delivered to the various points of use by a pipeline system. Very large cylinders are centrally stored in banks which automatically switch on to full cylinders when the cylinders in use become empty. Provided these cylinders are checked daily and the system is serviced regularly, this system makes for greater safety as there is very little chance of all the cylinders emptying unnoticed and the flow of gases failing.

Carbon dioxide absorbers
One of the problems of administering a general anesthetic is to ensure that the carbon dioxide being excreted by the patient is eliminated as fast as it is produced. One method of ensuring the elimination of this gas is to include a carbon dioxide absorber in the circuit. Though these absorbers may not be commonly used in Accident and Emergency departments where they are not important in the usual brief anesthetic, it is considered worthwhile to mention their use here. By using an absorber in the circuit, the anesthetic gases may be used at much lower flow rates, an aspect which is specially important in countries where medical gases are scarce and expensive. Further, the anesthetic gas can be used again and again provided sufficient oxygen is introduced into the circuit and, of course, the carbon dioxide is eliminated. Because of the reduced gas flows, less theatre pollution takes place.

The commonly used system is the circle absorber. The gases within the system travel round a circular route, controlled by unidirectional valves, and in this circuit a large canister containing soda lime granules is included. The expiratory valve for ridding the system of excess gases is situated either near to the patient or near the soda lime canister. Because of the large size of the granules only half the volume of the canister is occupied by the solid granules, the rest being occupied by air spaces through which the patient can breathe freely.

Soda lime, consisting of granules made up of calcium hydroxide, sodium hydroxide, potassium hydroxide and silicates, reacts chemically with, and thereby removes, any carbon dioxide with which it comes into contact. Usually soda lime changes colour as this chemical action occurs and alters the composition of the granules. A typical colour change is from pink, when fresh, to white when exhausted. When the colour change indicates that the soda lime is nearly exhausted it is discarded and replaced. In continuous use soda lime functions satisfactorily for several hours. As the soda lime reacts with the carbon dioxide heat is generated which can be felt by placing a hand on the canister.

It is important to note that trichloroethylene must never be used in association with soda lime because contact between the two produces toxic agents. Formerly it was common to use a simpler apparatus, the 'to-and-fro' (Waters) carbon dioxide absorber, which is described on p. 204 (and Figure 19.5).

Anesthetic circuits

The term 'anesthetic circuit' means the arrangement of tubing, reservoir bag and expiratory valve, by which anesthetic gases and vapours are delivered to the patient from an anesthetic machine. The nurse should know a little about the different types of anesthetic circuits because, in an emergency situation she may have to help an anesthetist during general anesthesia. Furthermore, she may find herself alone in the Accident and Emergency department having, on her own initiative, to use an anesthetic machine to administer oxygen to an accident victim (p. 227).

MAGILL CIRCUIT (Mapleson A – Figures 19.2–19.4)
Basically this consists of wide bore corrugated tubing with a reservoir bag attached to it, near to the anesthetic machine, and an expiratory valve situated near to the patient. Fresh gases enter the tubing from the anesthetic machine and pass freely to the patient. The gases enter the reservoir bag to fill it but should not distend it. As the patient inspires, he takes gases from the tubing and reservoir bag which, therefore, partly deflates. On expiration, the reservoir bag fills again, partly as a result of the patient's expiration and partly because fresh gases enter the system from the machine. Simultaneously excess gases leave through the expiratory valve. The flow of gases must be at least 7 l/min for an adult patient. A higher flow rate will not harm the patient but low flow rates will. The adequate flow of gases rids the circuit of excreted carbon dioxide. Failure to do this will lead to the detrimental effects of carbon dioxide accumulation (p. 163) – raised blood pressure and pulse rate and increased capillary dilatation, most noticeable to the observer as skin flushing.

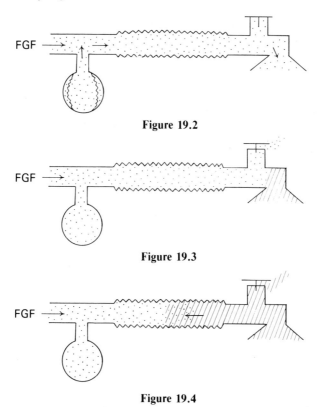

Figure 19.2

Figure 19.3

Figure 19.4

☐ Fresh gas   ▨ Alveolar gas   ▨ Mixture of fresh gas and alveolar gas

Figures 19.2–19.4 Composition of gas flow in Mapleson A circuit during spontaneous ventilation. **Figure 19.2** Inspiration; **Figure 19.3** Midway through expiration; **Figure 19.4** End of expiration

The expiratory valve consists of a very light, mobile circular plate which can move from its seating to allow gases to pass in one direction, but which returns to its seating when the gas flow stops, being aided by a light spring. The tension on this spring can be regulated by a screw arrangement on the top of the valve (p. 228). This valve is used wide open during spontaneous respiration to prevent resistance to expiration, which would be tiring for the patient and, in the conscious patient, would lead to a sensation of suffocation. It is adjusted to exert minimal resistance to expiration, just enough to prevent emptying and collapse of the reservoir bag. The valve is used closed or nearly closed when the patient has to be ventilated by intermittent manual compression of the reservoir bag (p. 227).

WATERS' CIRCUIT

In this system the reservoir bag is situated near to the patient and the expiratory valve (Figure 19.5). The supply of fresh gases enters the circuit between the valve and the reservoir bag. A Waters' soda lime canister may be placed in the circuit between the bag and the fresh gas supply but it is not as popular as it was in earlier years.

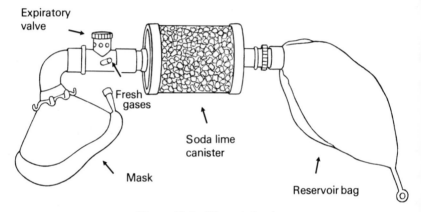

Figure 19.5   Waters' circuit

CO-AXIAL BREATHING CIRCUITS

In these circuits, gases are led to and from the patient by lightweight corrugated tubing which contains small bore tubing. The expiratory valve and reservoir bag are both remote from the patient, situated at the end of the corrugated tubing nearest to the anesthetic machine.

There are two co-axial systems in common use.

(1)   In the Bain circuit, the gases are delivered to the patient along the internal narrow tubing, and the expired gases flow back along the corrugated tubing, between it and the internal tubing.

(2)   In the Lack circuit, the fresh gases are led to the patient by way of the outer channel between the two concentric tubes while the expired gases return along the inner tube, which is much wider than in the Bain circuit, to the expiratory valve and the reservoir bag.

In both systems, the expired gases are channelled from the expiratory valve to a scavenging device. This may be a simple charcoal canister which removes the halothane vapour from the expired gases, or it may be an elaborate ducting system which sucks out the waste gases and vapours, and exhausts them to the atmosphere outside the hospital building.

20

Care before and after anesthesia

A. KILPATRICK

Preparation for out-patient anesthesia

The role of the nurse in preparing the patient for out-patient anesthesia is vitally important. In fact a strong case could be made out to demonstrate that her role is at least as important as that of her medical colleagues. She has earlier, more prolonged and constant contact with the patient, and it is at this stage that the patient's confidence in his many attendants can be established – or irrevocably shattered. The nurse who attends the patient from the time of his arrival at the hospital, whether as an emergency admission or by prior arrangement, has a strong influence on the patient's psychological attitude and responses. She has the opportunity to engender an air of quiet calm and confidence, which is more reliable than the effect of any anxiolytic drug, but this can be dispelled by careless talk in the patient's hearing. She must not be overheard discussing his condition. She may, of course, in response to the patient's questioning, discuss aspects of his condition or management which come within her ambit and knowledge. Similarly, the patient should not be able to overhear anyone discussing the clinical findings or the treatment of any other patient for two very sound reasons. First of all there is the question of confidentiality which prevents clinical or other details being conveyed, even accidentally, to another person. Secondly, a patient overhearing a discussion about another patient can quite easily and mistakenly believe that the details he has overheard refer to himself, with potentially disastrous results. Therefore, when the nurse is not speaking to the patient, or to a colleague in the course of her duties, she should follow the advice of the war-time poster 'Be like Dad, keep Mum'. Once the patient is settled into the Accident and Emergency department and the need for a general anesthetic is established, various procedures must be observed. The nurse will have responsibilities for part of them but she must have a little knowledge of them all.

HISTORY

The first procedure to be conducted by the anesthetist is the history taking, but prior to this the nurse may be able, from her early contact with the patient, to give helpful information to the anesthetist. He is interested in previous serious illness, anesthetic complications at previous operations, and concurrent drug therapy – some patients carry cards detailing their drugs and the dosages.

The patient's dental health is relevant. He may wear part or full dentures. Dental crowns are particularly vulnerable to damage during endotracheal intubation and the risk of damage can be minimized by prior knowledge. The presence of loose teeth is of interest, and this may occur both in children, when their deciduous teeth are soon to be lost, and in adults with a very neglected dentition.

A urine sample is examined for the presence of abnormalities which would give a clue to systemic disease. Sugar, albumin, blood and acetone are the principle abnormal constituents to be sought.

It is important for the anesthetist to be aware of his patient's mental state and the nurse's early observations can help here. Is the patient calm, apprehensive, excitable or even mentally unstable with a tendency towards violence which may be triggered off during the recovery period after the general anesthetic?

PHYSICAL PREPARATION OF THE PATIENT

(1) The patient should have had nothing to eat or drink for a minimum of 4 hours prior to induction of anesthesia. Problems arise in patients suffering from surgical shock which delays stomach emptying for much longer than usual. These patients may have a significant amount of gastric contents for much longer than 4 hours after their last meal or drink. It is the anesthetist's responsibility to decide when it is safe for him to administer the anesthetic, bearing in mind other factors involved such as the seriousness of the surgical condition – can it, for example, be safely left longer without detriment before attempts are made to correct the surgical complaint? A drink given 4 hours prior to anesthetic should not be a hypertonic glucose drink, as this may be retained in the stomach for an excessive time after ingestion. There is also a problem with children, especially young ones, who may suffer from dehydration if left for periods in excess of 4 hours without a drink.

(2) Dentures, artificial limbs, artificial eyes, spectacles and contact lenses should be removed before the patient is taken to the anesthetic room. Some doctors advise the removal of lipstick,

nail varnish and other cosmetics prior to anesthesia because these may mask any vascular changes in the skin.

(3)   The patient should be invited to empty his bladder before being presented for anesthesia. If he is unable to do so, and it is thought that his bladder may be full, his medical attendant may consider it advisable to catheterize the patient before or during general anesthesia.

(4)   An identification label must be fastened to the patient prior to going for his operation if he is to be admitted to a ward afterwards. This label should preferably be around a wrist or ankle where it should not interfere with the operation site. The label should be put on while the patient is conscious and can check the details. The information relevant to young patients under 16 years (18 in USA) or patients unconscious or dazed on arrival at the hospital should be checked with a responsible adult. The details should include the patient's name and his case record number.

(5)   Consent. Though it is the doctor's responsibility to obtain the written consent of the patient or his guardian, the nurse should check that this has been done before the patient goes to the operating area. If the patient is not in a fit state to give consent, a responsible adult should be asked to do so on the patient's behalf, after the significance and purpose of the operation has been explained to the person signing the form. Parental consent should be obtained for patients under 16 years of age (18 in USA). Such consent should be in writing though occasions may arise when this cannot be done because of the urgency of the operation. In these circumstances verbal consent given over the telephone by a parent or guardian to a responsible nurse or other member of the medical team may have to suffice.

PRE-OPERATIVE MEDICATION (PREMEDICATION)
Premedication refers to drugs given prior to an anesthetic to make the administration of that anesthetic easier for the patient and the anesthetist. The specific reasons for the use of premedication are:

(1)   To allay the patient's fear and anxiety before the proposed anesthetic and operation.

(2)   To reduce the secretion of saliva, whose presence would cause difficulties during the anesthetic. Saliva acts as a foreign material which can irritate the larynx and bronchial tree during the period of unconsciousness and cause coughing.

(3)   To prevent undesirable reflexes, such as cardiac arrhythmias, which may occur during anesthesia. These can be caused by

drugs such as halothane, trichloroethylene, and suxamethonium (succinylcholine).

(4) To play a part in the anesthetic technique itself. An analgesic
drug given as premedication provides some protective analgesic
effect during the operation.

(5) To produce some amnesia for the period immediately prior to
the operation. Various drugs such as diazepam and lorazepam
are used to produce amnesia.

It is common practice in ward situations when dealing with in-
patients, to give premedicant drugs by intramuscular injection 45
minutes pre-operatively. The out-patient may be dealt with differently
in that the anesthetist often gives a premedicant anticholinergic (parasympatholytic, see below) drug, and perhaps an analgesic drug, by the
intravenous route immediately prior to induction of anesthesia.

Premedicant drugs
Two anticholinergic (parasympatholytic) drugs commonly used in
premedication are atropine and hyoscine which are given as described
in the previous paragraph. These drugs have an inhibiting action on the
vagus nerve, blocking the parasympathetic effect on the heart (p. 126)
and protecting the heart from anesthetic drugs which might otherwise
produce cardiac arrhythmias. The patient may well be aware of his
increased pulse rate after the injection, especially if it has been given
intravenously. The secretion of saliva is inhibited, too, and the patient
will be aware that his mouth feels drier than normal. The production of
saliva is reduced because its presence in the mouth and pharynx during
anesthesia might lead to it acting as foreign material and irritating the
larynx, so causing a bout of coughing or laryngeal spasm.

While hyoscine may cause minimal drowsiness, atropine does not.
One or other drug, probably more commonly atropine, will be given to
all patients undergoing general anesthesia on an out-patient or in-
patient basis.

It will be realized that while there are a large number of drugs suitable
for premedication purposes, many are unsuitable for the out-patient
who will be taken home after he has recovered sufficiently on the
hospital premises. Nevertheless, the anesthetist has the ultimate
decision concerning which drug or drugs he wishes to use depending on
clinical circumstances, not the least of which will be the decision
whether or not the patient is to be admitted to hospital for 24 hours or
more after the operation. An Accident and Emergency department will
have patients who have only minor complaints which do not require
admission afterwards, and also patients suffering from major trauma
requiring prolonged in-patient treatment.

Narcotic analgesic drugs are often used as pre-operative medication in the ward situation, but seldom in the Accident and Emergency department. When given in this department they are most commonly given by the intravenous route to patients who will be admitted later to a ward for 24 hours or more. Their duration of action is too long for out-patient use as they leave the patient drowsy for 4 hours or more. Drugs in this group include morphine, papaveretum, pethidine (meperidine), and pentazocine. In addition, fentanyl can be included in this group. It reputedly has a much shorter duration of action and is given mostly by the intravenous route. Other drugs used for premedication purposes for in patients and mentioned here for completeness, are the sedative benzodiazepines, a typical example being diazepam, and the phenothiazines typically promethazine and trimeprazine. They all have a hypnotic effect too prolonged for routine use in out-patients.

Post-operative instruction for out-patients after general anesthesia
The lingering post-anesthetic effects vary from patient to patient and are affected by the drugs used for anesthesia, the general fitness of the patient and the age of the patient. One would expect an elderly patient to take longer to fully recover than a younger patient. However, in general the following instructions apply to all those being sent home soon after a general anesthetic.

The patient must be taken home in the care of a responsible adult but not left alone when home is reached. In other words, while the responsible adult may in some instances be an ambulance man rather than a friend or relative, the patient should not be taken to a residence where he will be alone during the next 24 hours or so. Once at home, the patient should rest there for the first 24 hours or until the next morning if that is near to 24 hours after the anesthetic. He must not get involved with cooking or hot kettles lest a hot pan or kettle of boiling water is spilled over himself or anyone else. The patient must not drive a car or cycle for 24 hours nor must he operate machinery during this period. No alcohol must be consumed as its intoxicating effect would be enhanced by any residual sedative effect of the anesthetic.

If it is anticipated that the operation site will be painful during the immediate post-operative period the patient may be given oral analgesic tablets to take when required. Such drugs would include one of the following depending upon the choice of the anesthetist and the anticipated severity of the pain: soluble aspirin, codeine, paracetamol (acetaminophen) or a paracetamol/dextropropoxyphene mixture, dihydrocodeine (drocode), diflunisal.

Diflunisal is reputed to have a 12 hour duration of action, hence it is to be taken only twice in a 24 hour period. The others may be taken at

4–6 hourly intervals. The tablets should not need to be taken more than four times in the day. The patient is recommended to adjust the timing of the dosage so that the last dose is taken at bedtime, before he settles down for the night. The reason for this advice is obvious as any pain tends to be more noticeable and distressing when the patient is trying unsuccessfully to sleep.

Before the patient's discharge home these instructions and warnings should be repeated to him and to his escort. The surgeon's instructions regarding care of a plaster cast or wound dressing should similarly be reinforced. The patient must, of course, be told that if any untoward symptoms occur he should either contact his own doctor or the Accident and Emergency department or perhaps even return to the department if telephoned advice seems inadequate or inappropriate.

21

Stages of anesthesia

F. WILSON

The nurse usually has difficulty in remembering the stages of anesthesia. However, they are very similar to those seen following the intake of alcohol. Consequently, she can always refresh her memory, even outside hospital, of the possible effects of anesthesia by recalling or observing the antics of the local population after partaking of wines and spirits or other alcoholic beverages.

In the comparison below, between a patient who is given an anesthetic and a person who has taken alcohol, rightly or wrongly the latter is referred to as 'the drunk'. His state is regarded as being due to 'alcoholic anesthesia' (intoxication). The condition of the patient receiving a gaseous anesthetic is referred to as 'general anesthesia'.

There are four stages of general anesthesia, namely: analgesia – stage 1, delirium – stage 2, surgical anesthesia – stage 3 and respiratory arrest – stage 4. As the patient is increasingly affected by the anesthetic his anesthesia is said to become 'deeper'. During recovery from anesthesia he is said to become 'lighter'. As anesthesia deepens he passes from stage 1 towards stage 4. As anesthesia lightens he passes from the state of surgical anesthesia (stage 3) towards stage 1 and the recovery of consciousness.

Alcoholic anesthesia (intoxication)	*General anesthesia*
Analgesia – stage 1	
The drunk walks into a tree, apologizes, walks away and is apparently unaware of the pain from his cut head. He is in a state of alcoholic analgesia.	Awareness of pain is the first sensation to diminish or disappear. This stage of analgesia is used in midwifery to reduce the intensity of labour pains. A 50% nitrous oxide – 50% oxygen mixture or a trichloroethylene inhaler relieves the pain but allows the patient to remain conscious and co-operative.

Delirium – stage 2

All parties start quietly. As the consumption of alcohol increases so does the amount and noise of the conversation. Eventually different reactions emerge. Some people become garrulous, others noisy, aggressive or affectionate. They are in the stage of alcoholic delirium. Afterwards they may claim to have been not responsible for their actions and blame them on the drink. Some, later, have no recollection of the events or conversation in which they were involved.

However, 'the quiet drinker', who constitutes the majority, drinks his alcohol and enjoys the effect without disturbing anybody. If he does take too much he goes to sleep without resorting to the antics of his noisy companions.

Many patients pass through stage 2 without causing any disturbance, but will remark that they dreamed as they were going to sleep. However, delirium often occurs and may manifest itself in several ways.

The patient may move his arms or legs, especially if he is trying to make himself comfortable. If movements are pronounced but are unlikely to cause damage to himself or to the nursing staff then those around him should take gentle hold of his limbs. The nurse allows her hands to move with the limb of the patient. After 2 or 3 minutes he usually settles down and becomes still. If, at this stage, she uses force to stop limb movement he may become violent and start to kick and strike out at all and sundry.

Violent reactions do occur spontaneously and it is then necessary to abandon the anesthetic or else use forceful restraint until deeper anesthesia is established.

Surgical anesthesia – stage 3

Further intake of alcohol causes unconsciousness and failure to respond to severe pain. In the cowboy films a bottle of whiskey is usually eagerly accepted and consumed by the victim prior to removal of a bullet or amputation of his limb – he is seeking surgical anesthesia.

At this stage the tongue loses its tone. Respiratory obstruction and

Stage 3 anesthesia is reached when the patient becomes unconscious, unresponsive to surgery and has regular respirations. Because some operations are more painful than others the anesthetist grades his depth of anesthesia accordingly.

During the stage of surgical anesthesia he protects the patient against respiratory obstruction.

Alcoholic anesthesia   *General anesthesia*
(intoxication)

Surgical anesthesia – stage 3 (continued)

regurgitation of stomach contents
can occur and cause fatal
asphyxia. Such an outcome is not
uncommon in acute alcohol
poisoning. The unconscious
drunk in hospital (or elsewhere)
should be placed on his side,
treated and observed as if unconsciousness were due to receiving a
general anesthetic.

Respiratory arrest – stage 4

Cerebral depression may be so
profound as to depress the
respiratory centre sufficiently to
cause respiratory arrest and
death.

Skilful administration of a
general anesthetic ensures that
respiratory arrest rarely occurs.
However, if it does the anesthetic
is discontinued and air or oxygen
is given by means of a resuscitation bag or anesthetic machine
until the patient becomes lighter
and spontaneous respiration
returns.

NURSING CARE DURING INDUCTION OF ANESTHESIA
Mind and body
The nurse tries to make the patient comfortable in mind and body.
Many patients are more afraid of the anesthetic than of the actual
surgery. They may be afraid that surgery will be started before they are
asleep, that they will wake up in the middle of the operation, not
awaken at all or that they will tell their innermost secrets as they are
coming round. Reassurance by the nurse does much to allay these fears.

Physical comfort is important whilst awaiting or during induction of
anesthesia. After emptying the bladder the patient is kept warm and the
elderly or breathless patient is given the choice of having his head raised
on two or three pillows.

Noise is kept to a minimum. Conversation during induction is best
restricted to that between patient and anesthetist. Sudden noise such as
the dropping of instruments or slamming of doors can startle the
patient and exacerbate his reactions when he enters the delirium stage of
anesthesia.

For several reasons the nurse should always remain with the patient during induction, maintenance and recovery from anesthesia. For example, her presence helps to reassure the patient. She can hold his hand and is available to restrain him during his stage of delirium. She may be needed to turn him into the head-down and lateral position if he threatens to vomit. Finally her presence as chaperone protects the doctor. Dreams occuring during anesthesia sometimes occur in the form of a sexual fantasy and as a result the doctor may be accused of assaulting the female patient.

Although attention has been drawn to loss of pain and consciousness it is important to know how hearing, swallowing and vomiting are affected by anesthesia.

Effect on hearing

Hearing is the last sensation lost before unconsciousness supervenes. Apart from a sudden noise exacerbating or initiating delirium, all those present must take care regarding what they say, in case the apparently unconscious patient can still hear. Although a remark made about the patient's size, state of cleanliness or temperament may be relatively harmless it can cause offence.

RECOVERY FROM ANESTHESIA

During recovery from anesthesia the patient passes through all the stages mentioned on the previous pages but in reverse order.

Hearing is the first sensation to return and discretion as to what is said is again important. Therefore, emergence from anesthesia should be allowed in quiet surroundings. Emergence delirium can be alarming. The author has been dragged out of the Accident and Emergency department into the street by a patient coming round from anesthesia who thought he was 'fighting for his life'. He has also been held by the lapels of his white coat by a once well known boxer who, quite wrongly, considered the anesthetist to be a worthy opponent! Personal damage can occur to patient, staff and surrounding property during emergence delirium. It is wise to allow the patient to take his own time to come round. Slapping his face to accelerate the return of consciousness is undesirable and may produce a profound reaction.

Prevention of respiratory obstruction and protection of the airway against the inhalation of vomit etc. are discussed in Chapter 17. His care on discharge from hospital after anesthesia is described on pages 210 and 211.

22

Intravenous anesthesia

F. WILSON

Surgical anesthesia is produced quickly by the intravenous injection of such agents as thiopentone (thiopental), methohexitone (methohexital) or a mixture of the two steroids alphaxalone and alphadolone. The Accident and Emergency nurse can do much to help both patient and anesthetist so that the patient remembers the way he is put to sleep, without fear, and perhaps even with pleasure.

Correct holding of the arm receiving the injection ensures the appearance of prominent veins, and thus a bigger target for the anesthetist, and minimal pain for the patient.

Technique

GRIPPING THE ARM

The function of gripping the arm is to make the veins conspicious. The nurse spreads out her thumb and forefinger to form an arch and with them applies pressure along their entire lengths thus forming a solid barrier across the thin walled veins. The target veins, usually in the antecubital fossa, that is at the front of the elbow, or on the back of the hand, should lie at the midpoint of the thumb–forefinger arch.

Any gap between the patient's arm and the nurse's grip, or having the target veins near the ends of her finger and thumb, may cause inadequate venous distension and possibly failure to achieve venous puncture.

Pressure of the grip is firm but not excessive. Too energetic application of pressure has the same effect as an arterial tourniquet, in that it cuts off the arterial supply so that the veins are unable to fill. This effect is most likely to occur in the young child or shocked patient. If in doubt as to whether she is gripping the arm too hard the nurse can confirm that she has not obliterated the arterial supply by feeling the presence of the pulse with her other hand.

SUPPORTING THE ARM
It is not unusual for the obese patient to occupy the whole width of the trolley (gurney) so that there is little or no room to rest the arms, whereupon he has to fold his arms across his chest. In these circumstances whenever antecubital vein puncture is anticipated it is customary for the nurse, in an attempt to present the veins for injection, to place her foot on the framework of the trolley, just above the wheels, and rest the prominence of the elbow upon her knee. Overextension of the elbow joint causes pain and should be avoided. Discomfort is also caused if the patient's arm is extended and pressed downwards over the poles in the carrying canvas on which he rests; they are best removed.

MAINTAINING THE GRIP
Many failures at venepuncture occur due to the premature release of the nurse's grip. Some doctors, rather than try to pass the needle through the skin and into the vein in one movement, prefer to pierce the skin and then redirect the needle into the vein. If she releases her grip after the first movement the veins collapse. In order to make the vein prominent again the whole procedure has to be repeated. The nurse should maintain her grip until asked to release her hold.

RELEASING THE GRIP
Releasing the grip when the needle is in the vein must be done by gentle relaxation of the nurse's finger and thumb. A careless, jerky release causes the tissues to jump at the needle point which then punctures the vein wall and spoils the whole procedure.

When an intravenous anesthetic is being given the patient may involuntarily move his arm. Usually he tries to flex his elbow or rotate his hand at the wrist. If movement is pronounced the needle may come out of the vein and cause an extravenous injection of anesthetic drug. The nurse avoids this, by releasing her grip gently and firmly clasping the patient's wrist to prevent movement until the injection is complete.

As the patient goes to sleep another involuntary arm movement may occur. Loss of muscle tone may cause the arm to bend at the elbow due to it sliding off the side of the trolley. The nurse prevents this, after releasing her initial grip above the antecubital fossa, by sliding the palm of her other hand under the elbow to keep the elbow joint extended. This support of the elbow and her hold on the wrist, as mentioned above, are maintained until the needle is withdrawn.

Painless–painful injections
Those who have been on the receiving end of injections, including doctors and nurses, are often surprised how painless or how painful

they can be, depending on the skill of the injector. Often the intravenous injection is the only thing the patient can remember about his anesthetic and on it he makes his judgement accordingly. Anesthetists are experts at intravenous injections and putting up transfusions, but a great deal of their success is due to the way the nurse holds the arm.

Although the above discussion is mainly directed towards the administration of intravenous anesthetics in many hospitals the nurse takes intravenous samples of blood. She should follow the same pattern when trying to enter a vein. One other factor remains. People are frightened of needles and the patient should be told when the needle is about to be introduced. The author always tells the patient to cough. As he obeys, the needle is simultaneously introduced through the skin. The cough is used to distract attention and is very useful in children. Penetration of the skin is the most painful part and should be quick and decisive. If, instead, the needle is advanced slowly intradermally, the patient quite justifiably complains of intense pain and the young child bursts into tears.

Intravenous anesthetics
Intravenous anesthetics act quickly. Unconsciousness occurs within 10–20 seconds of their administration. They are popular because the patient is subjected neither to the smell of a general anesthetic vapour nor to the application of a face mask.

On recovery from an intravenous anesthetic the patient passes through the stages of anesthesia described on p. 212. However, passage through the stages is so swift that the patient is unaware he has gone through the delirium stage, and has no time to dream or get excited.

Because, as regards time, the stages of anesthesia are compressed together, it is obvious that respiratory arrest can occur quickly and often without warning. Other undesirable events that can occur are respiratory obstruction, laryngeal spasm, vomiting and regurgitation. Therefore, it is of paramount importance that intravenous anesthetics should not be given unless there are available a portable resuscitation bag or anesthetic machine with the oxygen supply turned on and an anesthetic circuit correctly assembled, suction apparatus in working order, equipment for intubation and the patient resting on a tiltable trolley. At this point it is appropriate to remind the nurse that before any anesthetic is given, or before any unconscious patient is placed on a tiltable trolley he is so positioned that if he regurgitates or vomits (or threatens to) his head can be lowered by raising the foot end of the trolley. There is no time in such eventualities to reverse the position of the patient if he has been placed on the trolley the wrong way round.

DURATION OF ANESTHESIA
Intravenous anesthetics act quickly but recovery is also rapid. If

anesthesia needs to be maintained for more than 2 or 3 minutes the anesthetist gives further incremental doses or else introduces inhalational agents such as nitrous oxide and halothane (fluothane).

MUSCLE RELAXANTS
Suxamethonium (succinylcholine) is the muscle relaxant most often used in the Accident and Emergency department.

An intravenous, intramuscular or subcutaneous injection of suxamethonium completely paralyzes all voluntary muscles within 10–30 seconds. Included in the paralysis are the muscles of respiration and those in the vocal cords. Paralysis lasts from 2–10 minutes. Accordingly, all precautions must be taken to deal with the certain occurrence of respiratory arrest and also possible eventualities such as the relaxed tongue (p. 166) and regurgitation.

Use of suxamethonium (succinylcholine)
Because the vocal cords are the guardians of the larynx, they are very sensitive and react violently by going into spasm if touched by an endotracheal tube; hence they are first rendered unresponsive by analgesic cream, jelly or spray, deep anesthesia or by paralysis of their muscle fibres. Suxamethonium does the latter and enables the endotracheal tube to be inserted through the open cords without causing them damage.

A frequent question asked is, 'if suxamethonium lasts only for 2–10 minutes does the patient after this time respond to the presence of the tube by coughing or going into spasm?' The answer is divided into several parts. Briefly, the answer is 'yes' unless further precautions are taken. Therefore, the anesthetist, before performing the actual intubation, may spray the cords and the trachea below them with a 4%' lignocaine (lidocaine) local analgesic spray. Another method, often combined with the use of a spray, is to smear the lower end of the endotracheal tube with 2% lignocaine gel or 1% cinchocaine (dibucaine) ointment.

In these circumstances recovery of the muscle tone in the vocal cords allows them to move, but being insensitive they do not react to the presence of the endotracheal tube, provided it is not moved.

Another alternative to keep the cords unresponsive is to deepen the anesthesia so that they stay asleep like the rest of the voluntary muscles or to give additional doses of suxamethonium.

If the cords are not kept insensitive or paralyzed the patient starts coughing. The cords also go into spasm and although the presence of the tube prevents their approximation, and hence closure of the larynx, the bronchi too can react by going into spasm. The patient then stops breathing and may become cyanosed.

LACK OF SEDATION AND ANALGESIA

Muscle relaxants do not put the patient to sleep and do not relieve pain. This is why the conscious patient is given an intravenous anesthetic before the suxamethonium injection. If his condition demands prolonged muscle paralysis, as is achieved by incremental doses of suxamethonium or by the injection of a longer acting muscle relaxant such as tubocurarine or pancuronium, the patient is given a narcotic (p. 231) or an inhalational anesthetic to keep him unaware of his condition and his surroundings.

Insufficient dosage of narcotics or inhalational anesthetics during paralysis, following muscle relaxants, results in 'awareness', that is, the patient being aware of what is going on around him. He can hear, often see, and feel pain yet is unable to move because of his paralysis. He is unable to speak because of his flaccid vocal cords and the presence between them of the endotracheal tube. 'Awareness' is distressing, and should be avoided by the judicious administration of drugs, but in emergency situations it may be difficult to achieve instant relaxation and unconsciousness without undesirable cardiovascular depression.

The paralyzed patient on ventilator treatment in the Intensive Care Unit can often hear and is aware of his surroundings. Consequently those around should choose their words carefully in his presence.

If there is a possibility of 'awareness' the nurse talks to him as if he were awake, explaining that he is all right, but cannot speak because of the tube in his throat and that his voice will return when the tube is removed. The Accident and Emergency nurse is advised to visit the Intensive Care Unit nurse and see how she deals so effectively with the patient on a ventilator.

23

Artificial ventilation

F. WILSON

The Accident and Emergency nurse is often the first person to encounter the patient who is breathing inadequately, or who has stopped breathing completely. His life may depend on her ability to restore ventilation. She must therefore be familiar with the equipment used for performing artificial ventilation and also be capable of using it effectively. However, before these are discussed the nurse should know what is meant by intermittent positive pressure ventilation (IPPV) and be familiar with the appropriate apparatus.

Intermittent positive pressure ventilation (IPPV)
Whenever respiratory movements are unable to produce an adequate tidal volume (p. 142) and respiratory obstruction is not present, then artificial ventilation is performed by squeezing a bag and forcing the gas contained therein into the lungs. The lungs are inflated. Their expansion forces the ribs and muscles of the chest wall to expand outwards and the diaphragm to move downwards. When the pressure on the bag is released, the weight of the chest wall presses upon the underlying lungs so that the air within them is squeezed out, through a valve (p. 228) into the atmosphere. This phase of respiration is also assisted by the elasticity of the lungs which return to the position of rest they adopt during the expiratory phase (p. 150).

Because every inflation of the lungs is provided by applying positive pressure to the bag, this type of ventilation can be regarded as positive pressure ventilation. However, the bag is squeezed only to produce inflation whereas expiration occurs without outside help. Therefore, positive pressure is applied to the bag only intermittently. This intermittent inflation of the lungs due to squeezing a reservoir bag is known as Intermittent Positive Pressure Ventilation, which is abbreviated to IPPV.

Therefore the essential difference between normal spontaneous respiration and IPPV is that in the former the ribs and diaphragm move first and pull the lungs out to their inspiratory position, in IPPV the nurse, or mechanical ventilator, pumps air into the lungs so that the lungs move first, and push the ribs outwards and the diaphragm downwards.

APPARATUS FOR IPPV

The basic requirements for performing effective ventilation are (Figure 23.1):

(1) A supply of air or oxygen.
(2) A rubber bag – usually referred to as a reservoir bag, to enable the resuscitator to squeeze air or oxygen into the patient.
(3) A face mask (or endotracheal tube and connector).
(4) An expiratory valve to allow air or oxygen to escape to the atmosphere during the expiratory phase (p. 150) of respiration, i.e. when the lungs deflate.

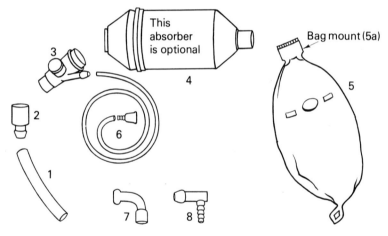

Figure 23.1   Circuit for performance of intermittent positive pressure ventilation (IPPV). Key:
　　　　1 Rubber tube which connects with endotracheal tube via a Nosworthy connector (7) or Rowbotham oral connector (8)
　　　　2 Catheter mount
　　　　3 Expiratory valve with feed (attachment for oxygen supply line)
　　　　4 Water's carbon dioxide absorber (canister)
　　　　5 Reservoir bag with bag mount (5a)
　　　　6 Air or oxygen supply tube for connection to air oxygen cylinder, pipe line or anesthetic machine
　　　　7 Nosworthy connector
　　　　8 Rowbotham connector

Apart from the face mask, which is detachable, all of these are provided as one unit in portable resuscitation bags such as the Ambu (p. 224 and Figure 23.2) or Air Viva. An alternative is to use a standard anesthetic circuit (Figures 23.5 and 23.6). The components of such a circuit should be collected and connected together so that all that needs to be done when the patient arrives is to turn on the oxygen supply, as in other circumstances it is too late to assemble pieces of apparatus when they are urgently needed.

Ventilators
The bag may be squeezed by hand or by mechanical means in the form of a 'ventilator'. Many different designs of ventilator are available, but basically they contain a bag, often shaped like a concertina, that encloses a volume of air, oxygen or anesthetic gas. When compressed the contents of the bag are thrust into the lungs. However, this positive pressure created in the lungs is maintained for only a second or so, after which the ventilator stops its pumping action. When sufficient inflation of the lungs has taken place a valvular mechanism in the ventilator allows the air, oxygen or anesthetic gas to escape. Simultaneously, the normal elasticity of the lungs and the weight of the chest wall squeeze air out of the alveoli, back through the ventilator and out into the surrounding atmosphere. After an expiratory phase (p. 150), whose duration is regulated by a setting on the ventilator, the next inflation of the lungs starts off a new respiratory cycle.

The mechanical ventilator can therefore act as another pair of hands. It is a robot but, just like the human being, it can go wrong. Occasionally it may stop without warning, develop a leak or perhaps continue its pumping without respite, even when it is doing harm to the patient. However, despite these undesirable possibilities, a ventilator is vital for long-term resuscitation procedures, and when used properly and observed carefully it is regarded as a hard working and much appreciated friend.

The Accident and Emergency nurse is unlikely to have to understand the full management of a ventilator because its use in her department is restricted. However, like her colleague in the operating theatre and Intensive Care Unit she must know what to do should the power fail in a ventilator being driven by electricity. In these circumstances she changes the lever, or levers, on the ventilator from 'automatic' to 'manual', whereupon she manually compresses the bag with her hands to maintain the IPPV in an identical way to that performed when utilizing the basic resuscitation circuit described on page 224.

IPPV WITH PORTABLE RESUSCITATION BAG (AMBU, AIR VIVA, ETC)
The portable resuscitation bag (Figure 23.2) has incorporated in it a

special type of valve called a non-return valve. As the name implies, the function of this type of valve is to allow all the air that is squeezed from the reservoir bag to enter the lungs, and to ensure that all the air breathed out by the patient is discharged into the atmosphere, thus avoiding the re-inhalation of stale air.

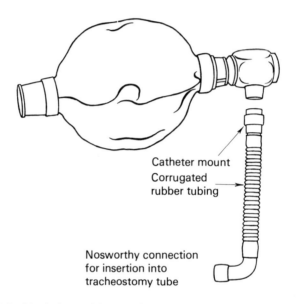

Catheter mount
Corrugated
rubber tubing

Nosworthy connection
for insertion into
tracheostomy tube

Figure 23.2   'Ambu' portable resuscitation bag. The valve is the non-return type

Squeezing the bag forces air into the patient. Releasing the bag allows him to expire through the valve into the atmosphere. At the same time the bag returns to its original shape, drawing into itself, through a separate entrance, a further supply of fresh air.

Protruding from the tail of the portable resuscitation bag is a nipple which can be connected, by means of a piece of rubber tubing, to a source of oxygen. If oxygen is introduced into the bag its flow rate is restricted to 1 litre/min. Higher oxygen flow rates will overdistend the bag and make it difficult to manipulate.

On first encountering the patient, the nurse invariably uses the bag with an attached face mask.

Technique of applying IPPV with resuscitation bag
  (1)   Acquiring an airtight fit between face and mask. The objective of squeezing the bag is to push air into the lungs. This cannot be

done unless the nurse acquires an airtight fit between the mask and the patient's face. Practice is necessary before she is able to claim success in every patient she attempts to resuscitate. She must keep the following actions in mind.

With her little, ring and fore fingers she elevates the chin (Figure 23.3), in order to draw the tongue away from the posterior pharyngeal wall thereby acquiring and maintaining patency of the airway.

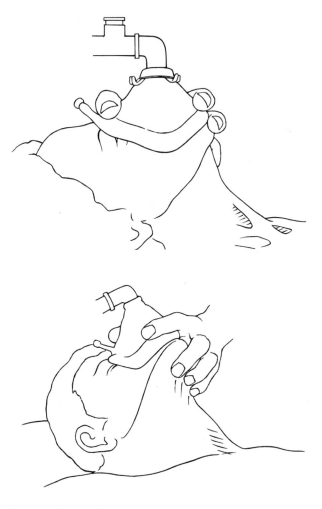

Figure 23.3   Applying mask to face – grip on mask and face

Her index finger is placed on the top of the lower front part of the mask and her thumb on the upper nasal part of the mask. Both of these digits press the mask firmly on to the face of the patient and establish an airtight fit. Therefore, the outer (lateral) three fingers apply pressure in exactly the opposite direction to the index finger and thumb. The nurse develops a balance between the two pressures so that when the bag is squeezed the contained air passes freely in and out of the patient's lungs.

She may have to alter the position of the head of the patient, either flexing it or extending it a little before she finds the one that is free of obstruction.

Sometimes even a skilled anesthetist finds it impossible to ventilate the patient satisfactorily especially if the patient is edentulous. If the nurse encounters difficulty in inflating the lungs of the patient she should insert an airway (p. 169). Usually this removes the cause of the difficulty which is frequently due to the respiratory obstruction caused by the relaxed tongue and lips.

(2) Connection to endotracheal tube. The nurse may find herself looking after a patient with an endotracheal tube in position who suddenly stops breathing. Without delay she has to start IPPV. She does this with the portable resuscitation bag, but she requires a catheter mount and a piece of corrugated rubber tubing to connect the bag to the endotracheal tube and its connector (Figure 23.4).

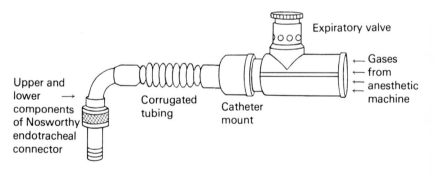

Figure 23.4   Catheter mount and endotracheal connector

(3) Squeezing the bag. The bag has a volume of 1200 ml (1.2 l). Because the tidal volume (p. 142) of an adult is between 450–600 ml it is obvious, if no leak exists, that the nurse has to

squeeze the bag sufficiently to reduce its size by half. There is no need to squeeze it so as to empty it completely. This may even do harm by producing excessive pressure within the chest and thus interfering with the return of blood to the heart (see below).

Technique of applying IPPV
With portable resuscitation bag the technique of applying IPPV is the same whether it is performed with a mask or by connection to the endotracheal tube.

The nurse should perform rhythmical compression and release of the reservoir bag, in such a way that the chest and abdominal movements resemble the movements and timing of the normal spontaneous respirations of the healthy resting patient. In this way she is more likely to produce adequate and satisfactory ventilation of the lungs. Therefore, over a period of 5 seconds the nurse performs IPPV as follows.

With the patient's chest in a position of expiration she starts slowly counting 1, 2, 3, 4, 5.

She counts 1	Inspiratory phase (p. 150 and Figure 16.6a and b)	During this period she squeezes the bag and thereby inflates the lungs.
She counts 2	End of inspiratory phase	She releases the bag.
She counts 3, 4	First part of expiratory phase	Expiration occurs due to the weight of the chest wall and the natural elastic recoil of the lungs.
She counts 5	Second part of expiration phase, i.e. expiratory pause.	The lungs are immobile.

The extent of the inflation of the lungs depends upon the degree of pressure which she applies to the reservoir bag. Too little expansion of the chest results in underventilation of the lungs. Overzealous compression of the reservoir bag creates too high a pressure within the patient's chest and prevents the return of blood to the heart. Reduction of the venous return to the heart prevents the heart from filling with blood so that when the atria and ventricles contract they discharge an inadequate volume of blood into the aorta and the blood pressure falls as a result of the diminished cardiac output (p. 124).

With an anesthetic circuit resuscitation is often performed using standard anesthetic equipment that is usually available on any anesthetic machine. Because many circuits are complex the nurse is advised to acquaint herself with two of the simplest types, both of which are perfectly suitable for routine IPPV (Figures 23.5 and 23.6). Both circuits incorporate a Magill-type expiratory valve (Figure 23.7) and the nurse must know its function, how it works, and how it is manipulated.

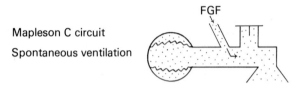

Figure 23.5   FGF – fresh gas flow (usually oxygen)

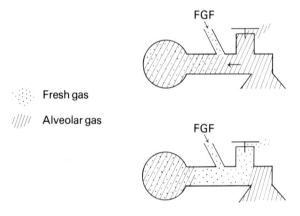

Figure 23.6   FGF – fresh gas flow (usually oxygen)

Circular disc – when turned clockwise closes valve. When turned anti-clockwise opens valve

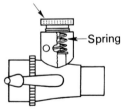

Figure 23.7   Expiratory valve

In circuit 1 (Figure 23.5) oxygen is received through the side lead directly from an oxygen cylinder, pipe line or from an anesthetic apparatus.

In circuit 2 (Figure 23.6) oxygen is delivered from the anesthetic machine.

In both circuits the flow rate of oxygen, as shown on the flowmeter, is set at 6 l/min. Both circuits can be attached to a mask, or connected to an endotracheal tube.

The nurse has to regulate the expiratory valve and squeeze the bag. Correlation in performing these actions needs practice. One suitable technique is as follows. First, the nurse turns on the oxygen supply at a rate of 6 l/min and applies the mask to the patient's face or connects the circuit to an endotracheal tube.

Action 1
She starts by screwing the valve in an anticlockwise direction until it is completely open. The reservoir bag fails to fill because all the oxygen escapes through the valve into the atmosphere.

Action 2
She screws the valve down by half a turn in a clockwise direction. The bag now starts to fill. When she squeezes the bag, its contained oxygen is forced out and has the choice of flowing into the patient or out through the valve into the atmosphere. To get into the lungs the oxygen has to do the work of distending the elastic lung tissue and lifting the overlying ribs and chest muscles. No such effort is required if it passes through a fully opened or almost fully opened valve. In these circumstances it is said that the resistance of the lungs and chest wall to inflation is higher than the resistance of the valve. With the valve fully open or almost fully open the oxygen takes the path of least resistance, it chooses to leave the bag and pass out of the valve into the external atmosphere. No oxygen enters the patient.

Action 3
The nurse now screws the valve down a further quarter of a turn in a clockwise direction. Turning the valve clockwise increases the tension or tightness of the valve spring so that oxygen finds it more difficult to escape into the atmosphere.

At this stage, compression of the reservoir bag results in some oxygen entering the lungs but most of it still leaks out of the valve.

Action 4
The nurse continues to screw the valve clockwise in quarter turns until eventually the resistance offered by the valve spring reaches a value which is approximately equal to that caused by the elasticity of the lungs

and weight of the chest wall. Oxygen can now enter the lungs or leave the valve with equal ease, and the nurse will find that compression of the reservoir bag produces movements of the chest wall that resemble a normal spontaneous inspiration.

Expiration takes place due to the normal elastic recoil of the lungs when the nurse releases the reservoir bag.

As when using the non-return valve in the portable resuscitation bag, she counts 1 as she squeezes the reservoir bag, releases on the count of 2, and allows the 3rd, 4th and 5th seconds for the lungs to empty.

At this point it is necessary to add a word of warning.

Care is taken to see that the valve is not screwed down fully, thus closing the escape routine completely, because all expired oxygen then returns through the absorber into the bag where it is joined by the fresh oxygen from the cylinder. Such a build-up of pressure in the circuit eventually causes a serious fall in cardiac output, and may burst the lungs and produce a pneumothorax.

It is repeated that to master such a technique takes practice. The nurse will find that she has often to adjust the valve by tightening or relaxing it a quarter of a turn one way or another. Eventually she will develop a 'feel' for what is going on in the patient's lungs. Lastly, but of great importance, at all times she must watch the extent and frequency of the respiratory movements of the patient, both of which are completely dependent on her skill in developing a liaison between her hands, the reservoir bag and the expiratory valve.

IPPV FOR THE CRUSHED CHEST

Crush injuries to the chest involving fracture of several ribs and/or the sternum usually need endotracheal intubation or tracheostomy followed by several days on a ventilator. A decision regarding the initiation of IPPV is easy in the severely ill patient, where paradoxical movements of the flail segment are obvious. However, it is sometimes difficult to decide what to do if the patient has two or three fractured ribs, even combined with some paradox, yet looks all right. In this type of patient, as in the more severely injured, it is important to measure PO_2 and PCO_2 (p. 237). The results are often unexpected and frightening. Breathing air may produce a PO_2 or 50–60 mmHg without any obvious distress to the patient. Repeated blood gas estimations are therefore essential over the next few days. Oxygen is given following the criteria discussed on p. 242. Any deterioration established clinically, or as a result of blood gas analysis calls for the introduction of IPPV, the purpose of which is to abolish paradox and improve ventilation.

Duration of IPPV is likely to last for up to 10 days. The short-acting suxamethonium is unsuitable for prolonged ventilation and is succeeded by longer acting muscle relaxants such as 30 mg tubocurarine or 6 mg pancuronium in the adult patient.

Precautions when using muscle relaxants
(1) *Lack of analgesia and sedation.* Muscle relaxants do not alleviate pain and do not put people to sleep (p. 220). Anaglesia and sedation are needed to relieve the pain and apprehension. In the adult patient the standard initial dose of analgesic is morphine 10 mg, papaveretum 20 mg, fentanyl 0.1–0.2 mg or phenoperidine 1–2 mg all of which are given intravenously. However, it is not unusual to give twice these amounts depending on the general condition of the patient. The first incremental dose of half the original dose may be needed within half an hour.

Often adequate dosage of analgesic is wrongly withheld because of the danger of respiratory depression. The latter does not matter because the respiratory movement of the patient is under the control of the ventilator.

Additional sedation is provided by benzodiazepines such as diazepam 10 mg intravenously or 10–20 mg intramuscularly, or a butyrophenone such as droperidol 2.5–5 mg intravenously. Incremental doses are half those given initially.

(2) *Dangers of positive pressure.* Whenever IPPV is started in the patient with chest damage the resuscitator must be on guard for the presence of a pneumothorax. If one is present and she intermittently forces air into the lungs she may be faced with a tension pneumothorax.

Therefore, at first, she squeezes the reservoir bag gently to inflate the lungs of the paralyzed patient. Inflation pressure is increased if there is no evidence of air leaking into the pleural space.

Some authorities automatically insert pleural drains with underwater seals in patients on ventilator treatment for chest injuries. This is because the sudden occurrence of a pneumothorax during IPPV can be fatal.

Obviously such pleural drainage is best performed before IPPV is commenced. However, if there is no time and the condition of the patient is desperate, it is essential to immediately insert an endotracheal tube with the restrictions applied to the inflation pressure as discussed above. Once control of the airway is established, a large bore needle or cannula is inserted into the pleural cavity to let out the air followed by more suitable drainage by catheter and underwater seal.

24

Partial pressure (tension) and blood gases

F. WILSON

The Accident and Emergency nurse should be familiar with the term partial pressure (tension) if she is to understand the significance of the blood gas readings which are so often quoted and discussed in modern medicine.

Partial pressure (tension)

The term partial pressure (tension) is usually abbreviated to P, the partial pressure of a gas in the alveoli is depicted P_A, and that in the arterial blood as Pa. These abbreviations however do not indicate which gas is being considered, and so the formula for the appropriate gas such as oxygen (O_2) and carbon dioxide (CO_2) is added as a postscript:

$\therefore$ P_AO_2 is the partial pressure of oxygen in the alveoli
P_ACO_2 is the partial pressure of carbon dioxide in the alveoli
PaO_2 is the partial pressure of oxygen in arterial blood
$PaCO_2$ is the partial pressure of carbon dioxide in arterial blood.

The Emergency nurse may then hear for example that the PaO_2 is low, the $PaCO_2$ is rising and IPPV must be started immediately. The next question is what exactly is meant by partial pressure? If the nurse finds difficulty in visualizing particles of gas she should imagine three men together trying to push a car with its brakes on. The total amount of push or pressure exerted on the car by their hands is equal to the sum of all the three individual pressures that they exert. However, each individual exerts only *part* of the total pressure exerted on the car; each man exerts a *partial* pressure which is the same amount of pressure he would exert if he were pushing alone. The same reasoning applies if the men are exerting their partial pressures on the inside, instead of the outside of the car, as if trying to escape from inside a police van on a Saturday night. Taking the analogy a step further, if all men were of equal strength but instead of three, there were 100 men consisting of 50

Englishmen, 30 Scotsmen and 20 Welshmen who were exerting pressure, it is easy to see that the English would exert 50/100 of the pressure, the Scots 30/100 and the Welsh 20/100. In other words the partial pressure exerted by each type of countryman would be in proportion to the number present of that particular nationality.

Returning to gases and replacing the men by gas particles and the car by the walls of an alveolus or the lining of a blood vessel, it is easy to understand why the partial pressure is defined as that pressure which a gas, in a mixture of gases, would exert were it alone. Furthermore, it helps to explain how the composition of the gases in the lungs and blood can be converted into partial pressures.

CONVERSION OF PERCENTAGE COMPOSITION TO PARTIAL PRESSURES (TENSIONS)

To do this it is necessary to recall that the air around us, i.e. atmospheric air, consists by volume approximately 20.9% oxygen, 0.04% carbon dioxide and 79% nitrogen (Table 16.9). Together, at sea level, they exert a pressure upon us of one atmosphere, which is capable of supporting a column of mercury (Hg) 760 mm high. The total pressure exerted by these three gases in dry air is therefore 760 mmHg. To find their partial pressures it is necessary to know (compare the men above) that each gas exerts a proportion or part of the total pressure according to whatever percentage of the total volume its particles occupy.

Therefore, because the total pressure exerted by the three gases is 760 mmHg and air consists of:

20.9% oxygen, the partial pressure exerted by the oxygen is

$$\frac{20.9}{100} \times 760 = 159 \text{ mmHg}.$$

Similarly the partial pressure of carbon dioxide in atmospheric air

$$= \frac{0.04}{100} \times 760 = 0.3 \text{ mmHg}.$$

At this stage it is important to realize that because inspired atmospheric air contains only a negligible amount of water vapour (0.06% partial pressure $\frac{0.06 \times 760}{100} = 0.45$ mmHg) it is regarded as being 'dry' air with no water vapour present.

PARTIAL PRESSURES (TENSIONS) IN THE ALVEOLI

The continuous exchange of gases between alveoli and pulmonary capillaries causes the alveolar air to contain less oxygen than air but more carbon dioxide than inspired (atmospheric or fresh) air. the volume percentage composition of alveolar air is approximately

oxygen	15.0
carbon dioxide	5.6
nitrogen	79.0
water	0.4

It is important to note that when the dry inspired air passes through the respiratory passages it picks up water vapour from the mucosal lining, so that by the time it reaches the alveoli it holds as much water vapour as it can and is said to be fully saturated. Now water vapour is a gas and so exerts a partial pressure which has been shown to have a value of 47 mmHg. Consequently, in alveolar air the oxygen, carbon dioxide and nitrogen together exert a pressure of one atmosphere minus the partial pressure of water vapour, i.e. $760 - 47 = 713$ mmHg.

At this stage it is necessary to recall that the 760 mmHg pressure in inspired air is exerted by dry gases, there is no water vapour present. In the alveoli, however, the pressure exerted by the dry gases is only 713 mmHg because 47 mmHg pressure is exerted by water vapour. This observation is important because when deriving partial pressures from percentage volumes of air it is customary to regard the total pressure as that exerted by the dry gases; the partial pressure exerted by the water vapour is excluded.

$\therefore$ In alveolar air the partial pressure of O_2 (P_AO_2) is

$$\frac{15}{100} \times 713 = 106 \text{ mmHg}$$

$$CO_2 \ (P_ACO_2) \frac{5.6}{100} \times 713 = 40 \text{ mmHg}$$

A P_AO_2 of 106 mmHg and a P_ACO_2 of 40 mmHg are regarded as normal values for a healthy person breathing air. If he breathes a higher percentage of oxygen than that in air his P_AO_2 will rise accordingly. For example, if he breathes pure oxygen his alveoli will contain their 'usual' 5.6% carbon dioxide, expelled from his pulmonary capillaries, leaving the remaining $100 - 5.6 = 94.4\%$ consisting of oxygen. This gives a

$$P_AO_2 \text{ of } \frac{94.4}{100} \times 713 = 673 \text{ mmHg}$$

If, on the other hand, the oxygen intake is reduced by hypoventilation so that its alveolar content is only 5% then the P_AO_2 is

$$\frac{5}{100} \times 713 = 35 \text{ mmHg}.$$

It is obvious, therefore, that provided oxygen can get or be got into the alveoli the higher the oxygen concentration breathed, the higher will be the P_AO_2. Similarly, if the patient is breathing air but is hypoventilating, the CO_2 will be retained in the alveoli, the P_ACO_2 will rise and the P_AO_2 will fall.

Provided that the nurse follows the concept of partial pressures in the alveoli, it only remains to show how they influence the partial pressures of oxygen (PaO_2) and carbon dioxide ($PaCO_2$) in the arterial blood.

PaO_2 AND $PaCO_2$

That a gas can exert a pressure in a liquid is obvious when the cap is removed from a bottle of lemonade or when a can of soda water is punctured. The bubbles of gas escape because they are previously confined in the container at a pressure greater than atmospheric. They escape until the pressure of carbon dioxide in the container is equal to that in the atmosphere. When the pressure of CO_2 in the container and the atmosphere are equal no more CO_2 escapes from the liquid – the lemonade or soda water is now 'flat'. In other words a state of equilibrium is reached. Similar events happen when the gases in the alveoli come into close contact with the blood in the pulmonary capillaries, they are separated only by a thin and permeable membrane. As a result the oxygen passes into the blood because the alveoli have a higher partial pressure of oxygen than the blood entering the pulmonary capillaries. Transference of the oxygen from alveoli (P_AO_2 = 106 mmHg) to pulmonary capillary blood is rapid, within 0.75 seconds, and almost complete equilibrium is reached. The result is that the blood leaving the lungs has an oxygen partial pressure of 103 mmHg. This blood is then returned to the heart, discharged into the aorta and can be sampled in, for example, the femoral or radial arteries (p. 236). Such a sample can provide the partial pressure of oxygen in an artery and hence it is referred to as the PaO_2. Because a little blood which has not passed through the lungs enters the heart the PaO_2 usually has a value of 100 mmHg in the healthy young adult, rather than 103 mmHg as would be otherwise expected. Therefore, there is only a little difference of 6 mmHg in such a person between the P_AO_2 and the PaO_2.

Similarly, the partial pressure of CO_2 in the blood entering the pulmonary capillaries, being higher than that in the alveoli, causes it to move out into the alveoli to be exhaled. The blood leaves the lungs with a carbon dioxide partial pressure ($PaCO_2$) equal to that in the alveoli (P_ACO_2), which in the normal healthy person is equal to 40 mmHg. The blood leaving the lung capillaries passes to the heart and into the arteries such as the femoral and radial, and a sample taken from these arteries gives the partial pressure of carbon dioxide ($PaCO_2$).

Measurement of PaO₂ and PaCO₂

Measurement of PaO_2 and $PaCO_2$ involve arterial puncture. Both examinations are derived from the one sample, which also fortunately provides other values such as pH (p. 245) bicarbonate (HCO_3) and base excess, all of which are known as acid–base readings which may help the clinician in his diagnosis.

Blood may be taken from any artery, but the most accessible are the radial, brachial and femoral. The radial and the brachial arteries are more difficult to puncture because they are smaller than the femoral, but the latter has the disadvantage that it is adjacent to the femoral vein which may be punctured in error.

Special precautions are needed for arterial puncture:

(1) The 2 ml syringe is heparinized as follows: 0.25–0.5 ml of heparin solution containing 1000 Units/ml is aspirated into the syringe, and the plunger withdrawn to the 1.5 or 2 ml mark. The syringe is rotated to spread a thin layer of heparin over its inner surface. The excess heparin is then discharged from the syringe by fully depressing the plunger. If more than a smear of heparin is left inside the syringe its acidity gives rise to false acid–base readings.

(2) Arterial puncture is painful and a small amount of local analgesic from a separate syringe is first injected around the artery. Too large a volume however may obscure the artery and make subsequent puncture more difficult.

(3) A 21 G × 3.8 cm (1.5 in) needle is attached to the 2 ml heparinized syringe and the plunger fully depressed before attempting arterial puncture. At all stages during aspiration of the blood sample air must be prevented from entering the syringe, because its gaseous content would alter the arterial blood gas readings due to the interchange of gas between the air in the syringe and the gases in the blood. The entry of air bubbles into the syringe is usually avoided if the plunger is withdrawn slowly.

(4) The technique of arterial puncture is different from that of venous puncture. In the former it is often easiest to transfix the artery with the needle. This means that the needle is first pushed right through the artery and then slowly withdrawn. As the needle point enters the artery the blood enters the syringe.

If during attempted introduction the needle touches but does not enter the artery, spasm immediately closes the lumen and makes it difficult to enter. The operator may then have to wait several minutes before the artery to relaxes.

(5) If a cannula is inserted, which enables further specimens to be

taken, it is necessary to heparinize the cannula by injecting 2 ml saline containing heparin through it every hour. An appropriate strength of heparinized saline is obtained by adding 5000 units of heparin to 1 l of normal saline.

Special care is needed if a three-way tap is attached to the cannula. If it becomes detached the patient may bleed to death, because the blood shooting out of the cannula at a BP of 120 mmHg will result in loss of blood similar to that from an unclamped cut artery of similar size.

(6) After removal of needle or cannula firm pressure is applied continuously for 10 minutes through a pad of wool or gauze – the nurse should not remove the pad to see if the bleeding has stopped before 10 minutes have passed, otherwise bleeding may restart. When bleeding has ceased a firm pad is secured by adhesive strapping over the puncture site.

(7) In most hospitals the blood sample, still in the syringe with needle attached (to restrict contact with air via the hub of the syringe), is taken immediately to the blood gas analyzer which provides a readout of the required examination within 1–2 minutes.

If there is ready access to such an analyzer, a plastic syringe can be used for taking the blood sample. If however the sample has to be transported down long corridors or to another hospital, or examination of its contents is delayed for other reasons, then a glass syringe should be used. Furthermore, it must be kept in the refrigerator when awaiting transportation and carried to its destination surrounded by crushed ice.

Blood gases

The PaO_2 and $PaCO_2$ are the values sought when the doctor asks for the 'blood gases'. They are however, considered in conjunction with the pH of the blood (p. 245). Diagnosis and treatment may depend on the PaO_2, $PaCO_2$ and pH values and although the Intensive Care nurse needs to be fully conversant with their normal values and their response to treatment, the Accident and Emergency nurse too will find them useful and interesting.

A few examples will show why this is so, but before abnormalities are considered it is necessary to return to and appreciate what happens if a normal patient is breathing air, oxygen enriched air or 100% oxygen.

When a normal patient breathes air the partial pressure of oxygen in his alveoli, P_AO_2, is 106 mmHg and the partial pressure of oxygen in his arterial blood, PaO_2, is 100 mmHg. Because these two values are approximately equal both P_AO_2 and PaO_2 will in future be regarded as having a value of 100 mmHg. The P_AO_2 and PaO_2 value of 100 mmHg remains normal, provided that the air gets to the lungs, takes part in adequate exchange with the blood and is discharged into the atmosphere, that is if there is normal ventilation. Another important factor is that the alveoli must be served with an adequate blood supply through the pulmonary capillaries which bring the carbon dioxide for elimination and collect oxygen to take back to the tissues. It is easy to see that disruption of the blood supply to the lungs can upset the balance between the alveolar air and the gaseous contents of the pulmonary capillaries, and therefore of the entire cardiovascular system.

POSSIBLE PROBLEMS
Apnoea (absent breathing)
If we hold our breath no gaseous exchange occurs between the alveoli and the atmosphere. The effect is that more and more oxygen is taken from the alveolar air and from the arterial blood so that the P_AO_2 and PaO_2 fall. Carbon dioxide accumulates in the arterial blood and the alveoli because it cannot escape and the P_ACO_2 and $PaCO_2$ rise. Arterial puncture would show a PaO_2 'say' of 70 mmHg (normal 100 mmHg) and a $PaCO_2$ of 60 mmHg (normal 40 mmHg). Hypoxia and carbon dioxide retention (termed hypercapnia or hypercarbia) are therefore present.

After 1–1½ minutes the urge to breathe becomes irresistible, largely due to the accumulation of CO_2 which stimulates the respiratory centre in the medulla. The effect is that the apnea is replaced by deep rapid breathing which quickly restores the PaO_2 to 100 mmHg and the $PaCO_2$ to 40 mmHg.

Blood gas readings similar to those found in voluntary apnea would be obtainable if taken from an unconscious patient whose tongue has been allowed to obstruct his pharynx. If however, the obstruction is not removed the PaO_2 falls to around 20 mmHg and the $PaCO_2$ rises to above 50 mmHg, and the patient dies because his respiratory efforts are unable to overcome the obstruction.

Hypoventilation
Between the above examples of the voluntary apneic person and the patient with complete respiratory obstruction there are those who have some degree of ventilation but it is below normal (hypoventilation). For example, sedative overdosage depresses brain function, including the response and activity of the respiratory centre. The effect is that the respiratory excursions are diminished and the $PaCO_2$ and P_ACO_2 rise, but in such a patient the depressed respiratory centre cannot increase the depth and rate of respirations. As a result the CO_2 accumulates in

the blood and because its partial pressure in the alveoli (P_ACO_2) rises, there is less 'room' for the oxygen and the P_AO_2 falls. Although the patient at first is suboxygenated according to his blood gas estimations (there is hypoxaemia), his tissues may still be provided with sufficient oxygen for their needs so that they continue to function and the patient remains uncyanosed. Eventually, however, as hypoxia and carbon dioxide retention (hypercapnia, hypercarbia) increase, the patient, if untreated, does deteriorate, oxygen lack becomes more pronounced and the patient dies.

The hypoventilating type of patient responds favourably to inter-mittent positive pressure ventilation (IPPV) with air or oxygen by means of a resuscitation bag, or if intubated, by means of a ventilator. IPPV flushes out the alveoli, washing out the CO_2 and replenishing the oxygen so that the P_ACO_2 and $PaCO_2$ fall and the P_AO_2 and PaO_2 rise. Such ventilation must continue until the patient has recovered suffic-iently for him to adequately ventilate his lungs unaided.

Arterial blood gas estimations in the Accident and Emergency department give valuable information as to the severity of hypoventil-ation and its response to treatment. Its use is not restricted in this context to the hypoventilation due to sedative overdosage for it is equally useful when investigating the effects of underventilation due to chest injuries (p. 230) or poliomyelitis or polyneuropathies (p. 268).

Shunts

If the entrance to an alveolus is blocked by sputum, inhaled fluid, inflammation or a growth but its capillaries remain open so that blood continues to pass through them, several disturbances occur regarding the interchange, or rather the lack of interchange, of gases between the blood and the alveoli. Blockage of an alveoli quickly results in all the oxygen being absorbed and the eventual collapse of the alveolar cavity, and hence no longer participates in gaseous exchange. Therefore, the blood supplied to it by its pulmonary capillaries passes by without getting rid of any of its CO_2, and without picking up any O_2. This unchanged blood is returned to the arteries of the general (systemic) circulation and is said to have been 'shunted' past the alveolus. A shunt thus refers to blood which has been returned to the aorta without passing through ventilated areas of the lung. The shunted blood mixes in the pulmonary veins with blood leaving areas of the lung which are ventilated, but the result is that the unaltered shunted blood prevents the PaO_2 from reaching its normal 100 mmHg. It may therefore fall to around 60 mmHg or less whereupon the hypoxia actually stimulates the respiratory centre whose subsequent increased activity tries to improve ventilation. But this has no effect on the shunted blood passing through areas of unventilated lung and so the PaO_2 remains low. However, the increased rate and depth of ventilation wash out the alveolar CO_2 so that the P_ACO_2 and $PaCO_2$ fall. Therefore, the combined presence of a low PaO_2 and low P_ACO_2, when the patient is breathing air, suggests the presence of a shunt, such as occurs following chest trauma, infection, drowning, or the inhalation of vomit.

Effect of breathing 100% oxygen
NORMAL PATIENT

Administration of 100% oxygen alters the composition of the alveolar air so that it consists of oxygen, carbon dioxide and water vapour. The main effect is that the oxygen replaces the nitrogen which is present when the patient breathes atmospheric air. If the P_ACO_2 is 40 mmHg and the P_AH_2O (the partial pressure of water vapour in the alveoli) is 47 mmHg, then the P_AO_2 is:

$$760 - (40 + 47) = 760 - 87 = 673 \text{ mmHg}$$

If the patient is breathing normally or is being ventilated properly, and there is normal gaseous exchange between the alveolus and its capillaries, then the blood leaving the capillary will have a partial pressure of approximately 673 mmHg, which it almost maintains during its journey to the limb arteries where an arterial sample is taken and the PaO_2 is measured. In actual fact a little suboxygenated blood from the heart veins empties into the arterial blood (an example of a normal minor shunt) and has the effect of lowering the PaO_2 to about 660 mmHg. For descriptive purposes blood with such a PaO_2 can be regarded in non-medical terminology as 'superoxygenated'.

HYPOVENTILATING PATIENT

If a patient with a low PaO_2 and a raised $PaCO_2$ due to hypoventilation (p. 156) is given 100% oxygen and he is ventilated by means of a resuscitation bag or ventilator so that his respiratory excursions are normal, the effect is to raise his P_AO_2 to 673 mmHg. Provided the alveoli are patent and supplied by capillaries so that normal exchange of gases occurs between them, the PaO_2 rises to 660 mmHg. If, however, some of the blood is shunted past a non-aerated alveolus then the capillary in question cannot 'pick up' any of the rich oxygen supply of the alveolus and so the suboxygenated blood is returned to the arteries in its original state. It, therefore, mixes with the highly oxygenated blood from the capillaries which has traversed the walls of the oxygenated alveolus so that a mixture of 'superoxygenated' and suboxygenated blood enter the systemic arteries, having a PaO_2 considerably less than the 660 mmHg of the 'superoxygenated' blood. Hence there is a different response when a marked shunt is present in that even if 100% oxygen is given the PaO_2 can never reach 660 mmHg. This fact is used diagnostically, in that if a patient with a low PO_2 and deficient respiratory movements is given 100% oxygen, and his PaO_2 rises to around 660 mmHg the cause of his trouble is hypoventilation of patent alveoli. If however the PaO_2 only manages to reach 600 mmHg then his troubles are partly due to a shunt. In actual fact the effects of the shunt may be so dramatic that the PaO_2 may read as low as 50 mmHg even when being ventilated on 100% oxygen. Such a patient is very ill indeed.

To summarize

(1) A hypoventilating patient with patent alveoli when properly ventilated with 100% oxygen will raise his PaO_2 to around 660 mmHg.
(2) A patient with a shunt, even when properly ventilated with 100% oxygen, will not raise his PaO_2 to around 660 mmHg.

Already it can be seen that arterial blood gas estimations can contribute towards diagnosis, and help in assessing the effectiveness of treatment in the Accident and Emergency department, both of which are necessary if the facilities of an Intensive Care Unit are not immediately or are only remotely available. PO_2 estimations can be made repeatedly and usually only take a few minutes to obtain, especially if arterial cannulation has been performed.

From the fact that the PaO_2 depends to a great extent on the inspired oxygen concentration it is essential that the inspired oxygen concentration is recorded in the notes beside any PaO_2 reading. For example if a patient has a PaO_2 of 100 mmHg with an inspired oxygen concentration of 21%, that is when he is breathing air, he is obviously well as far as his pulmonary gaseous interchange is concerned. If however his inspired oxygen concentration is 100% and his PaO_2 is 100 mmHg he is seriously ill.

Further information may be obtained; for example, the response to treatment is indicated by the PaO_2 readings. A patient with a shunt, being ventilated with a constant oxygen concentration, and having a PaO_2 of say 150 mmHg is obviously improving if his PaO_2 rises to 200 mmHg and deteriorating if the PaO_2 falls to 120 mmHg.

At this stage it is well to remember that high oxygen tensions (partial pressure) in the blood may cause oxygen toxicity, and in fact can damage the lungs. Therefore, if a patient with a low PaO_2 is given oxygen, the PaO_2 should only be allowed to rise slightly higher than the normal 100 mmHg. If for example 100% oxygen raises the PaO_2 to 200 mmHg the percentage of oxygen can be reduced to 80% by increasing the percentage of air in the inspired mixture. If the PaO_2 still remains high, the percentage of air is gradually increased until the required PaO_2 is obtained. It is unusual to have to have a patient on 100% oxygen for more than a few hours.

Indications for giving oxygen

Many more patients come to harm when denied oxygen than if they are given oxygen.

The initial administration of oxygen is usually beneficial to the patient. Only occasionally does it do harm, and the Accident and Emergency nurse should never hesitate to use oxygen in the patient who is either breathless, cyanosed or comatose.

The response of the patient to receiving oxygen depends on whether he is accustomed to breathing in response to a higher $PaCO_2$ than is usual. This is explained as follows: the normal patient starts to breathe deeper and quicker if the carbon dioxide tension ($PaCO_2$) of his blood rises. However, in some lung diseases, such as bronchitis (p. 266) with emphysema and fibrotic diseases such as silicosis and pneumoconiosis, there is impaired gaseous interchange between the alveoli and their capillaries due to blockage of some alveoli by mucus and actual destruction of others due to the disease process. This results in the lungs becoming less efficient and the $PaCO_2$ tends to rise. Faced with this rising $PaCO_2$ the respiratory center often adapts and begins to respond to a $PaCO_2$ only at a higher level, perhaps a $PaCO_2$ of 50 mmHg. In these circumstances a sudden rise of $PaCO_2$ above 50 mmHg would still stimulate the respiratory center, which improves ventilation by increasing the rate and depth of respiration.

If the disease progresses slowly the $PaCO_2$ gradually rises to reach 70 mmHg which again is accepted as normal by the respiratory center. However there comes a time, usually when the $PaCO_2$ reaches this level of 70 mmHg, when the respiratory center cannot respond to any further rise in carbon dioxide tension. As the disease progresses further, the $PaCO_2$ still continues to rise and the respiratory center responds, but this time because of the reduced oxygen content in the blood. The stimulating factor, therefore, has changed from the raised $PaCO_2$ to the lowered PaO_2. This reduced PaO_2, by stimulating the respiratory center, improves ventilation and prevents the $PaCO_2$ from rising and the PaO_2 from falling further. Thus the patient's breathing mechanism depends on him having a lower than usual oxygen tension in his blood. If the PaO_2 is artificially raised by giving oxygen by face mask or nasal catheter the effect is to remove the hypoxia but at the same time it also removes the hypoxic stimulus to the respiratory center. The result is that he stops breathing and his $PaCO_2$ starts to rise. But the respiratory center cannot respond to a raised CO_2 tension and eventually the $PaCO_2$ reaches a level which causes loss of consciousness: he then has a CO_2 narcosis which soon proves fatal if not remedied by means of artificial ventilation.

To make the picture even more complicated a further factor is involved, namely the degree of hypoxia. Although hypoxia provides the stimulating drive to the respiratory center it only does so if the oxygen shortage is not severe. If hypoxia is pronounced the respiratory center itself suffers from oxygen lack, becomes depressed and the patient dies.

To summarize

A raised $PaCO_2$ stimulates the respiratory centre until the $PaCO_2$ reaches about 70 mmHg.

The hypoxia then takes over and stimulates the respiratory center, but if hypoxia becomes too severe the respiratory centre fails; 100% oxygen given to this type of patient removes the hypoxic drive leading to apnea and a fatal rise in $PaCO_2$.

TREATMENT

At first glance it may appear dangerous to give oxygen to certain patients, but it must be understood that hypoxia is more dangerous than carbon dioxide retention and must be relieved as soon as possible. Therefore oxygen must be given but the aim is to reduce the hypoxia from the level which depressed the respiratory centre to a level which stimulates it. Often this can be done by slightly increasing the oxygen from the 21% found in atmospheric air to around 24% or 28% with the use of an oxygen mask. This small amount of extra oxygen may elevate the PaO_2 sufficiently to decrease the hypoxia yet be insufficient to depress the hypoxic drive effect on the respiratory centre. This level of oxygen concentration is usually used in the wards until the antibiotics have had time to work and the patient coughs up his sputum and improves his gaseous exchange. The response of such a patient can be seen by his improved color and general condition or by estimation of his PaO_2.

Unfortunately every patient does not improve sufficiently on a slightly increased oxygen intake, especially if he is unconscious when it is then necessary to give him a higher oxygen intake, and because the treatment of hypoxia is an emergency he is usually given 100% oxygen. If his respirations fail he must be artificially ventilated by means of a resuscitation bag and mask or endotracheal tube and, according to individual preference, possibly through a carbon dioxide absorber (p. 204). This IPPV with 100% oxygen reduces or removes the hypoxia in most patients and the increased manual or mechanical ventilation washes out his CO_2 and returns it to normal levels. Removal of secretions by endotracheal or endobronchial suction may then improve the access of gases to the alveoli, so that he is soon able to maintain his own ventilation and gaseous exchange.

The percentage of oxygen in his inspired gases may then be reduced from 100% until it is eventually replaced by atmospheric air.

The Accident and Emergency nurse should never hesitate in giving a high percentage of oxygen to a patient who is semi-comatose or comatose. Usually he will improve dramatically. If he does not and continues to make apparently good respiratory movements there is little else she can do. If he stops breathing she must ventilate him artificially by means of a bag and mask until the doctor arrives.

Inspired oxygen concentration – oxygen mask
Several different oxygen masks are available. They deliver different oxygen percentages according to their design and to the amount of oxygen that is fed to them.

The Ventimask is available in five types which deliver 24, 28, 35, 40 or 60% oxygen when fed with oxygen at the rate stated on the mask.

The Edinburgh mask where the percentage of oxygen delivered depends on the oxygen flow rate which is fed into the mask.

Oxygen flow rate (l/min)	*% delivered from mask*
0.5	22–25
1.0	24–28
2.0	27–31
3.0	29–41

The MC mask delivers 40–50% oxygen when its oxygen supply is 4–8 l/min.

The mask from the anesthetic machine. If used, the oxygen supply should be regulated to deliver 6–8 l/min.

It is stressed that the Accident and Emergency nurse will rarely be confronted by a patient who responds unfavourably, that is becomes apneic, when given oxygen. Usually he is a bronchitic but even if he does stop breathing the nurse is able to ventilate him until the medical staff take over his resuscitation. In all other conditions where oxygen is necessary she should not hesitate to administer it either by oxygen mask or anesthetic machine. Many lives are saved, very few are lost (and none should be) by giving oxygen.

25

pH

F. WILSON

Everybody knows that vinegar has an acid taste. Fortunately acids can be detected without the need to taste them because they turn litmus paper red. Every acid has a formula. Vinegar, whose other name is acetic acid, has the formula CH_3COOH. Carbonic acid, the most important acid found in the blood, has the formula H_2CO_3 which can be written $H.HCO_3$. In both these formulae:

C is the abbreviation for carbon
O is the abbreviation for oxygen
H is the abbreviation for hydrogen

It can be seen that these and other acids have a single H component that is an H atom, at either the end or the beginning of the formula, as indicated by the arrows.

$$CH_3COOH$$
$$H.HCO_3$$

These particular Hs and *no* other in the formula detach themselves from the rest of the formula and are responsible for the amount of acidity in a solution. If many Hs split off the solution is said to be a strong acid and if only a few split off the solution is a weak acid.

Two important developments result when the H detaches itself. First it changes its name to 'a hydrogen ion'. It is written as H^+. Second, because the acid H has split off, the rest of the formula is 'non-acid' but it too changes its name, and the non-acid part of the formula is renamed the 'base'. Therefore, acetic acid splits up or dissociates into hydrogen ions and a base (which in this example is called acetate). Carbonic acid splits up or dissociates into hydrogen ions and a base (which in this example is called bicarbonate.) These splittings up or dissociations are written:

$$CH_3COOH \rightleftharpoons H^+ + CH_3COO^-$$
$$H_2CO_3 \rightleftharpoons H^+ + HCO_3^-$$

(For significance of arrows see p. 247)

It has been stated that the strength of an acid depends on the hydrogen ion (H^+) concentration. This expression is abbreviated to the symbol $[H^+]$.

pH: its meaning and relationship with $[H^+]$*

'p' stands for the power of something, and so pH (measured on a scale from 1–14) is another way of expressing the power or strength of the hydrogen ion concentration. pH is described as being equal to the negative logarithmic value, to the base 10, of the hydrogen ion concentration, which is written:

$$pH = \log_{10} \times \frac{1}{\text{hydrogen ion concentration}}$$

$$= \log_{10} \times \frac{1}{[H^+]}$$

Even if the nurse is unfamiliar with logarithms she can still understand much of the acid–base balance if she regards pH as being equal to $\frac{1}{[H^+]}$ provided she realizes that $\frac{1}{[H^+]}$ is a fraction. This is important because it explains why it is that when the H^+ ion concentration goes up the pH goes down. In order to explain this 'anomaly' it is necessary to appreciate that the mathematicians have been at work, and although they are experts at simplification they can cause problems to those who find the manipulation of numbers difficult. However, numbers can be manipulated to suit the manipulator. For example:

(1) Take the number 3
    Double it and it becomes $3 \times 2 = 6$ which is obviously greater than 3
(2) Take the number 3
    Divide it into 1 and it becomes the fraction $\frac{1}{3}$
    Double the original 3 so that the fraction becomes $\frac{1}{3 \times 2} = \frac{1}{6}$
    which is less than $\frac{1}{3}$. Therefore, as the original number 3 goes up the value of the fraction $\left(\dfrac{1}{\text{the original number}}\right)$ becomes less.
(3) Now substitute 'hydrogen ion concentration' $[H^+]$, for the original 3 in the fraction $\frac{1}{3}$ which becomes
    $$\frac{1}{\text{hydrogen ion concentration}} \quad \text{or} \quad \frac{1}{[H^+]}$$

*H^+ refers to a hydrogen ion. $[H^+]$ indicates the concentration of hydrogen ions.

It can be seen by the same reasoning as before that as the hydrogen ion concentration goes up the pH falls.

There are many acids produced in the body and they influence the degree of acidity of the blood. Usually the body eliminates quantities of acids which either it does not need or which would be harmful. Sometimes the body cannot dispose of the unwanted quantities of acids as quickly as it would like. Then, the acidity of the blood rises and the pH falls below the normal value of 7.4. If the acid level rises too much it becomes harmful and if treatment is not instituted the acid level, that is the hydrogen ion concentration, eventually proves fatal.

CARBONIC ACID

There are many acids in the blood. Carbonic acid (H_2CO_3) is produced when carbon dioxide is hydrated, that is when it combines with water. The reaction is symbolized as:

$$CO_2 + H_2O \longrightarrow H_2CO_3 \qquad \text{(Reaction 1)}$$

The H_2CO_3 then breaks up or dissociates into hydrogen ions (H^+) and bicarbonate ions (HCO_3^-):

$$H_2CO_3 \longrightarrow H^+ + HCO_3^- \qquad \text{(Reaction 2)}$$

These two reactions can be combined

$$CO_2 + H_2O \longrightarrow H_2CO_3 \longrightarrow H^+ + HCO_3^-$$

On the other hand the reaction:

$$CO_2 + H_2O \longleftarrow H_2CO_3 \qquad \text{(Reaction 3)}$$

means that carbonic acid can break up or dissociate or reconvert into carbon dioxide and water.
And, H^+ can reunite with HCO_3^- to form H_2CO_3:

$$H_2CO_3 \longleftarrow H^+ + HCO_3^-$$

$$\text{(Reaction 4)}$$

The four reactions may be combined as:

$$CO_2 + H_2O \rightleftharpoons H_2CO_3 \rightleftharpoons H^+ + HCO_3^- \quad \text{(Reaction 5)}$$

Arrows pointing in both directions indicate that the reaction can move either to the left ($\leftarrow$) or to the right ($\rightarrow$).

Reaction 1 suggests that if more CO_2 is produced then more H_2CO_3 is also formed making the blood more acid. This is in fact what happens in the body. Therefore, if the carbon dioxide tension ($PaCO_2$) rises so does the H_2CO_3 and this in reaction 2 produces more hydrogen ions (H^+). Because the hydrogen ion concentration [H^+] rises the pH falls.

The patient is said to be acidotic. Because the acidosis is principally due to increased CO_2 concentration due to abnormal respiration, the acidosis is said to be respiratory in origin – the patient has a respiratory acidosis. His $PaCO_2$ will be raised above 40 mmHg and his pH reduced to below 7.4.

If a person overbreathes, either voluntarily or due to fear, he washes out his CO_2. His $PACO_2$ falls and so therefore does his $PaCO_2$. Returning to the combined reaction 5, if CO_2 is lowered the H_2CO_3 tries to produce more CO_2, so some of it is used up in doing so. When the H_2CO_3 level falls the hydrogen ions (H+) and bicarbonate ion (HCO_3^-) are also partly used up trying to replenish the H_2CO_3. The effect is that the hydrogen ion concentration [H+] falls and so does the acidity of the blood – it becomes more alkaline; there is an alkalosis and because it is respiratory in origin it is known as a respiratory alkalosis: the $PaCO_2$ is lower than the normal 40 mmHg and the pH is raised above 7.4. Respiratory alkalosis is found in hysteria and in the first stage of salicylate poisoning.

Hydrogen ions (H+) are produced by other acids such as those found in excess in diabetes. Because the excess hydrogen ions (H+) produce an acidosis, but their increase is not primarily due to a respiratory disturbance, it is termed a non-respiratory acidosis or metabolic acidosis as it is due to a disturbance in metabolism. The pH is below 7.4.

The body tries to get rid of the excess hydrogen ions (H+) by overbreathing, in an attempt to excrete the CO_2 and hydrogen ions (reaction 4 followed by 3 – see also reaction 5) so that the $PaCO_2$ falls. The fall in $PaCO_2$ however is insufficient to restore the pH to normal (7.4). The result is that:

(1) the pH still remains less than 7.4 – there is a metabolic acidosis
(2) the PCO_2 falls trying to produce a respiratory alkalosis to counteract the metabolic acidosis, and restore normality to the acid–base status of the blood.

A patient with such a combination is said to have a primary metabolic acidosis with a compensatory respiratory alkalosis.

Many combinations of variations in PCO_2 and pH can occur, and in conjunction with the PaO_2 an accurate diagnosis can often be made in the Accident and Emergency department, and immediate treatment started.

Further reading

Wilson, F. and Park, W. G. (1980). *Basic Resuscitation and Primary Care* (Lancaster: MTP Press)

Jones, E. Sherwood (1978). *Essential Intensive Care* (Lancaster: MTP Press)

26

The unconscious patient

M. B. McILLMURRAY

Consciousness is a state of awareness which allows us to respond appropriately to others and to our surroundings. Consciousness may be altered by injury or illness, the type and severity determining the degree of alteration. This may be slight, the patient being drowsy, but easily rousable, or marked with the patient deeply unconscious and unresponsive.

The depth of unconsciousness can be determined by simple clinical assessment and may be arbitrarily divided into four levels as follows:

Level I   – Patient is rousable
Level II   – Patient responds purposefully to a painful stimulus
Level III – Patient responds in a purposeless fashion to a painful stimulus
Level IV – Patient does not respond to any painful stimulus.

The painful stimulus can be a squeeze of the Achilles tendon, in which case a purposeful response would be the withdrawal of the leg. A purposeless response might be a movement of all limbs, while the patient would remain motionless in the absence of a response. Observations of this sort, done repeatedly, give a relatively crude measure of the clinical progress of an unconscious patient.

In any unconscious patient the overriding priority is the maintenance of an unobstructed airway. The patient is best nursed in the lateral position with the head down, the neck extended and the chin held forward (see Figures 17.1 and 17.15). Dentures should be removed and an airway may need to be inserted to prevent the tongue blocking the throat; an endotracheal tube is sometimes preferable (p. 187). Excessive mouth secretions or vomit should be removed, preferably by suction, a process which may need repeating. Having established that the patient is breathing and there is a radial pulse, attention can be directed towards the cause. The Accident and Emergency nurse can greatly assist the doctor by obtaining as much information as possible from relatives, friends, police, ambulancemen, from the contents of the patient's pockets or handbag, records of previous hospital admissions and from examination of the patient. She may ask the following questions: Is this an accident victim? Is there a history of diabetes, epilepsy, depression, or hypertension? Was the unconsciousness sudden in onset or has it developed over hours or days? Were there syringes, drugs or empty drug bottles in the house or near the patient when he was found? Is there a suicide note?

Useful physical signs which she may observe include injection marks, body temperature, superficial injuries, focal neurological abnormalities, pupillary asymmetry, neck stiffness, and the smell of ketones on the breath.

The various more common causes of unconsciousness may be considered as follows:

(1) Transient with complete recovery likely and where no other treatment is necessary, for example:
     minor head injuries – concussion
     most drug overdoses
     epilepsy – the post-ictal state.

(2) Complete recovery likely once treatment is given, for example:
     diabetic ketoacidosis
     hypoglycaemia
     some drug overdoses
     epilepsy – status epilepticus
     hypothermia.

(3) Recovery possible, but usually delayed and may be incomplete, for example:
     severe head injuries
     strokes – including subarachnoid hemorrhage.

These disorders and their management are discussed below.

Head injury
Any patient who suffers a period of unconsciousness after a head injury, no matter how trivial, must be carefully assessed and observed from a neurological standpoint. This usually means admission to hospital for at least 24 hours. The unconsciousness which follows will vary in depth and duration according to the severity of the injury. The degree of recovery is variable, but usually complete. When unconsciousness is prolonged, it is essential to maintain hydration and nutrition; to attend to the processes of excretion and to avoid complications, notably infections, which may threaten the patient's life. The general aspects of supportive care are not discussed.

More immediate life-threatening complications develop if a blood vessel has been ruptured by the injury, for the ensuing hemorrhage and hematoma increase the pressure within the skull which is unable to expand to accommodate the increased volume. This rise in intracranial pressure is most serious when a meningeal artery is damaged. This event is usually accompanied by a skull fracture, the blood entering the extradural space. Surgical intervention is essential or death will rapidly ensue. Holes are drilled into the skull on either or both sides of the midline and the extradural hematoma is evacuated.

The signs of a rapid rise in intracranial pressure are:

(1) Deepening level of unconsciousness.
(2) Pupil asymmetry, with the pupil dilating on the side of the hemorrhage.
(3) Rise in blood pressure.
(4) Slowing of the pulse.
(5) Rise in body temperature.
(6) Appearance of focal neurological signs, including an extensor plantar response (positive Babinski's sign) on the opposite side to the hemorrhage.
(7) Blurring of the optic discs as seen with the ophthalmoscope.

Thus, the nurse will understand the vital importance of monitoring, at least once every 15 minutes, the pupil size, level of consciousness, pulse rate, blood pressure, and temperature in any patient who is or has been unconscious after a head injury. Urgent medical attention is essential if any of the signs of rising intracranial pressure develop. If both pupils become dilated and will no longer constrict in response to light, then irreversible brain damage can be assumed to have occurred.

A ruptured intracranial vein may only become apparent some time after the head injury. The typical story is of unconsciousness with recovery after the initial event, and a slow relapse into unconsciousness, the patient having complained of headache and vomiting after a variable latent interval. Blood oozes into the subdural space and surgical evacuation of the hematoma will effect a cure. The physical signs are similar to an extradural hematoma, though much less dramatic and there is usually more time to establish an accurate diagnosis.

Strokes

A stroke, alternatively known as a cerebrovascular accident or CVA, is the sudden cessation of blood supply to a part of the brain, the clinical effects depending upon the part affected. The blood flow may be interrupted by a blood clot, either a locally formed thrombosis, or an embolus from elsewhere, or by hemorrhage from a ruptured blood vessel into the brain substance. There is frequently a history of hypertension or heart disease, or in the case of younger females of taking the oral contraceptive. The commonest presentation is with loss of function and/or sensation down one half of the body, on the opposite side to the CVA. The affected limbs are initially limp (flaccid) and later stiff (spastic) and immobile, and the tendon reflexes become exaggerated with an extensor plantar response. Speech and comprehension are lost when the dominant cerebral hemisphere (the hemisphere controlling 'handedness' – i.e. the left in right-handed individuals and vice versa) is involved. This may give the erroneous impression of an altered level of consciousness, though the ability to hear and understand the spoken word is often retained. When consciousness is impaired, it generally indicates a large intracerebral hemorrhage or the development of intracerebral edema. Recovery in these circumstances is unlikely and even with surgical evacuation of the blood or treatment of the edema with steroids, permanent disability is virtually inevitable.

In an uncomplicated stroke, the defect is usually worst at the outset and recovery takes place to a variable degree over a variable period of time. The blood pressure is frequently raised initially, probably as a compensatory mechanism, but only rarely should it be treated at this stage. If the muscles of the pharynx and esophagus are affected, then swallowing may be difficult and aspiration into the lungs and infection are likely. Regular suction of secretions and nasogastric feeding will be required until recovery takes place. Patients are often very frightened especially when their powers to communicate are impaired, and they need great patience and understanding.

Rupture of a blood vessel into the subarachnoid space may occur in isolation or as an extension of an intracerebral hemorrhage. Consciousness may not be impaired in the absence of brain tissue damage, the patient typically complaining of severe headache, photophobia, vomiting and neck stiffness. Any forced movement of the head is extremely painful and the neck is rigid. Straight leg raising, likewise, stretches the meninges and is limited and painful. The diagnosis may be rapidly confirmed by passing a needle into the subarachnoid space below the lower end of the spinal cord, when blood-stained cerebrospinal fluid will be withdrawn. Initial treatment is sedation, pain relief and blood pressure control (if raised). Contrast X-rays of the carotid and vertebral arterial systems are performed at a later stage to determine the source of the hemorrhage – usually an intracranial aneurysm, with a view to surgery and the prevention of another bleed.

Self-poisoning

Self-poisoning is an increasingly popular form of attempted suicide and may be difficult to recognize if the patient arrives unconscious at the Accident and Emergency department. The majority, however, are conscious and frightened and will readily admit to their actions (p. 92). The drug (or drugs) must be identified either by examination perhaps with the help of the hospital pharmacist, or by contacting the patient's general practitioner. Analysis of stomach contents or screening of the patient's blood for various drugs may be necessary. With the exception of self-poisoning by corrosive agents, such as Lysol, which is instantly recognizable by the characteristic smell and the white, sloughed mucosa in the mouth and pharynx, a stomach washout should be attempted in all cases (p. 274). A large bore soft rubber tube is passed over the tongue down the esophagus and into the stomach with the patient held down and lying on his side. A funnel is inserted into the end of the tube and the stomach is emptied by allowing the funnel to drop into a bucket on the floor. The funnel is then raised to a level above that of the patient and a litre of tepid water is run in. The procedure is then repeated until the liquid coming back is clear, when the rubber tube may be withdrawn. This must *not* be attempted on an unconscious patient without first passing a cuffed endotracheal tube, otherwise there is a serious risk of aspiration of fluid into the patient's lungs. The treatment, thereafter, depends upon which drug has been taken. The more popular ones, which demand a particular course of action, are discussed below.

It is essential to recognize that self-poisoning may be attention seeking as well as a form of self-destruction. Therefore all patients are assessed later by a psychiatrist and the truly suicidal such as those with a recent bereavement, a history of depression and old age are selected for more specific treatment.

PARACETAMOL (ACETAMINOPHEN)

This drug is particularly dangerous because the effects of overdose do not appear for several days. They are dose-related and liver cell damage occurs which may be fatal. Biochemical evidence of liver cell damage appears 12–36 hours after ingestion. Fulminant liver failure may occur at 3–6 days with deepening jaundice, coma and kidney failure. Estimation of the plasma paracetamol level must be made immediately for, with the knowledge of the time interval between ingestion and blood sampling, it is possible to predict the degree of liver cell injury with some accuracy. N-Acetyl cysteine 150 mg/kg diluted in 5% dextrose given intravenously over 15 minutes, followed by 50 mg/kg in 500 ml of 5% dextrose infused over 4 hours, and a further 100 mg/kg in 1 l of 5% dextrose given over the next 16 hours, may prevent liver damage, but only if treatment is given within 8–10 hours of paracetamol ingestion.

DISTALGESIC (DARVON)
This is a compound containing paracetamol and a narcotic analgesic, dextropropoxyphene hydrochloride (propoxyphenehydrochloride). The latter may cause coma, convulsions and respiratory depression. Repeated small doses of naloxone, a specific narcotic antagonist, may be required to maintain respiration. Otherwise, the approach is the same as for paracetamol.

ASPIRIN
The clinical manifestations of salicylate poisoning include rapid breathing and pulse rate, sweating, deafness, and tinnitus. Consciousness is not impaired except as a pre-terminal event. Oral fluids should be encouraged in patients with mild poisoning, but with plasma concentrations above 50 μg/ml, a forced alkaline diuresis should be carried out. This is a way of promoting the excretion of aspirin through the kidneys by increasing the urine flow and changing the urinary pH to a level at which the drug will more easily dissolve. The procedure should be carried out in the intensive care unit because careful control of fluid, acid–base and electrolyte balance is essential.

CARBON MONOXIDE
Carbon monoxide combines with hemoglobin and prevents it from performing its function as a carrier of oxygen to the tissues of the body. The highest possible concentration of oxygen should be given without delay and in severe cases this may have to be administered in a hyperbaric oxygen chamber.

BARBITURATES
The clinical features of overdose include drowsiness, hypotension, hypothermia, respiratory depression and coma. The most accurate assessment of the respiratory effects is provided by the arterial oxygen and carbon dioxide concentrations (p. 235), though simple measures of tidal volume (p. 142) may also be useful. Artificial ventilation should be started if the arterial oxygen, that is the PaO_2, falls below 60 mmHg (p. 238). Hypotension is rarely marked and does not require specific treatment, apart from intravenous fluids when there is evidence of poor tissue perfusion (p. 134) as indicated by a falling urine output. The excretion of phenobarbitone and barbitone is enhanced by a forced alkaline diuresis (see above).

TRICYCLIC ANTIDEPRESSANTS (e.g. AMITRIPTYLINE)
These drugs are toxic to the heart. Disturbances of heart rhythm are common, and vary from a simple increase in heart rate to more serious and life-threatening abnormalities, including asystole. These are more likely to occur in patients with heart disease. Cardiac monitoring is essential in all patients for at least 24 hours, the rhythm abnormalities being treated in the usual way. Other effects include convulsions, urinary retention and coma.

Diabetes mellitus

Carbohydrates are the main source of energy for all tissues of the body and we cannot survive without them. They are metabolized, first to glucose, then either to glycogen, the form in which they are stored in the liver, or to carbon dioxide and water in the peripheral tissues, releasing in the process the energy which feeds the various cellular functions of the body. Insulin, a hormone liberated into the blood-stream from the pancreas, regulates these processes, and keeps the blood glucose concentrations within a narrow range throughout the day and night.

Diabetes mellitus is a functional disorder of the pancreas, in which insulin is produced in inadequate amounts, and occasionally not at all. Although there is plenty of glucose in the blood, there is inadequate insulin present to 'take it' into the tissue cells which are therefore starved of glucose. The body tries to increase the cellular glucose content by using other sources of energy such as fat and muscle protein. The patient becomes thin and weak with a rise in blood glucose concent-ration, and glucose appears in the urine. Large volumes of urine are voided to excrete the glucose in solution and the patient complains of excessive thirst. Eventually, a state of dehydration is reached and the body electrolytes are profoundly disturbed. The increase in fat metabolism produces ketoacids in amounts which exceed the capacity of the liver to dispose of them. They accumulate in the blood and appear in the urine, and the odour of acetone is noticeable on the patient's breath. The plasma bicarbonate concentration is reduced and a metabolic acidosis slowly develops (p. 248). The respirations increase in rate and depth and the alveolar carbon dioxide tension (P_ACO_2) falls. The patient lapses gently into unconsciousness (hyperglycemic or diabetic coma). At this stage the muscles of the alimentary tract are atonic, the stomach dilates with liquid and there is a danger of vomiting, with aspiration of the stomach contents into the lungs, and finally death, an avoidable terminal event in what must be regarded as a reversible disorder.

HYPERGLYCEMIA – HYPERGLYCEMIC (DIABETIC) COMA
The diagnosis of diabetic coma is normally obvious, especially in a

known diabetic. A history of thirst, polyuria and weight loss may be obtained from relatives or friends. The patient is dehydrated, with a fast pulse, low blood pressure and cold extremities. The breathing is slow and deep with the unmistakable smell of acetone on the breath. Urine, if obtainable, is loaded with glucose and ketones. Evidence of an infection, a frequent precipitating cause of coma in a diabetic, may be found. Treatment is directed towards rehydration, and blood electrolyte, pH (p. 246) and glucose control. Careful, frequent observation and regular measurements of the various biochemical parameters are essential because aspiration of stomach contents, fluid overload, potassium imbalance, and acidosis are the main causes of death in diabetic coma, but are all preventable or reversible.

Venous blood is taken for measurement of glucose, urea, and electrolytes. An arterial sample (p. 236) is analyzed for pH, $PaCO_2$, bicarbonate content and base deficit. A cannula is placed into a vein and an infusion of fluid and electrolytes is given at a rate dependent on clinical circumstances, but often as much as 4 litres are needed in the first 3 hours. A nasogastric tube is passed and the stomach contents are aspirated. Insulin is introduced, preferably through a second intravenous line by means of a continuous slow infusion syringe pump at a rate of about 8 units per hour, but varied according to subsequent blood glucose results. The patient should be attached to a heart monitor as the shape of the tracing gives an early indication of serious swings in plasma potassium concentration. If acidosis is severe, a bicarbonate solution is included in the intravenous fluid regime; potassium is invariably required at some stage and often in large quantities. Bladder catheterization is avoided if at all possible because of the danger of introducing infection. Further details of management are not discussed because the patient is rapidly transferred from the Accident and Emergency department to the Intensive Care Unit.

HYPOGLYCEMIA – HYPOGLYCEMIC COMA

Of more danger to the diabetic is the coma of hypoglycemia, a consequence of insulin excess. The brain relies entirely on glucose for its source of energy and if the blood level falls too low, the central nervous system becomes first excitable and then greatly depressed. Irreversible damage or death may follow untreated hypoglycemic coma and treatment before the diagnosis is established is justified. The early symptoms of hypoglycemia include trembling, sweating, hallucinations and irrational behaviour. All diabetics should be warned of the significance of such symptoms, as any sugar containing food or drink at this stage will prevent progression to the more serious problems of convulsions and coma, when intravenous glucose will be necessary. The Accident and Emergency nurse may be presented with the patient already unconscious and the distinction from hyperglycemic coma may be difficult. In hypoglycemic coma, the patient is generally well hydrated and sweating, respirations are not laboured and no acetone is detectable on the breath. The pupils may be dilated, the limbs flaccid with depressed or absent reflexes, and the plantar responses may be extensor. Blood is taken for sugar estimation and this is immediately followed by a 50 ml intravenous bolus injection of 50% dextrose. Improvement may be dramatic and consciousness may be restored before the injection is finished. Slower recoveries are treated with a continuous intravenous infusion of dextrose in a general medical ward. Adjustments to the insulin dosage are clearly necessary in the long term. If in any doubt about the cause of coma in a diabetic an intravenous injection of 50% dextrose is mandatory for it will have little effect in the patient who turns out to be hyperglycemic yet will be life-saving in the hypoglycemic patient.

Epilepsy

Epilepsy results from an intermittent electrical fault in the cerebral cortex of the brain. In its most dramatic form, a convulsion occurs in which the victim falls unconscious without warning and enters a tonic phase where the muscles are rigid, the teeth tightly clenched and the eyes rolled upwards. This may be accompanied by a loud cry, cyanosis, congestion of the face and engorgement of the veins. After a short time the clonic phase appears, in which there is a generalized shaking of trunk and limbs, frothing at the mouth and urination, which then slowly subside leaving the patient still and sleeping. The convulsion may only last a few minutes, but the unrousable sleep which follows may continue for several hours. Thus the nurse may only see this post-ictal state. It is important to distinguish the post-ictal state from other causes of unconsciousness and when a history is available this is easy. The patient has a normal colour, though breathing is laboured. The limbs are limp, reflexes are lost and the plantar responses extensor. Pupils are dilated and may not respond to light. No treatment is necessary, apart from the usual attention to the airway.

If a convulsion is witnessed in the Accident and Emergency department it is usually best to allow it to run its course. There is no point in attempting to restrain the patient and the time is probably better spent in pacifying other patients who may be very frightened by the incident. During the clonic phase there is a risk that the patient's tongue may be injured between clenched teeth and if possible a gag should be inserted between the jaws. Under no circumstances should the nurse's fingers be used for this purpose.

Rarely, convulsions may occur repeatedly without restoration of consciousness between them. This is called status epilepticus and is a medical emergency because brain anoxia will occur unless they are controlled. Various anticonvulsant drugs are now available such as phenytoin, sodium valproate and carbamazepine, but a continuous intravenous infusion of diazepam is considered the most suitable method of managing this situation. The dose which is used is adjusted to give complete fit control, whereupon consciousness will eventually be restored and adjustments made to the patient's previous oral preparations.

Other forms of epilepsy such as, petit mal, temporal lobe and focal epilepsy, are unlikely to present in the Accident and Emergency department and are therefore not discussed here.

Hypothermia
Exposure to cold for a prolonged period slows body processes and results in unconsciousness and death. The very young and elderly in the winter are especially vulnerable. There is usually evidence of self-neglect and the patient has often not been missed for several days before being found at home in poorly heated surroundings. The body is cold to the touch, respirations are depressed and may be scarcely noticeable. The pulse is slow and the blood pressure hard to find. Reflexes are diminished and slow in response. The diagnosis is established by recording the rectal temperature with a low-reading thermometer. Temperatures of 29 °C are not unknown. The possibility of some underlying disorder must be considered. For example, a patient sustaining a stroke may be unable to summon help and be found several days later; and more rarely, an underactive thyroid gland, resulting in hypothyroidism, may present in this way. The latter is of some importance, for recovery in that instance will only take place if appropriate thyroid replacement treatment is given. In general, treatment consists of slow rewarming ('space' blankets are useful for this purpose) and intravenous hydration is usually necessary because raising the temperature is a lengthy process. Death is common, despite these measures, and complications such as acute pancreatitis are not infrequent.

27

The patient with chest or esophageal pain

M. B. McILLMURRAY

The importance which is attached to the complaint of chest pain comes from the knowledge that 1 in 5 of all deaths in this country are from a myocardial infarction (heart attack). Yet, only a small proportion of patients presenting to the Accident and Emergency department with chest pain will have had one. Thus, this section first briefly considers the ways in which the various causes of chest pain can be distinguished from one another, and then the problem of heart attacks in more detail.

Great emphasis is based upon the patient's description of his chest pain. Typically, the pain of myocardial infarction is a severe, crushing sensation felt anteriorly in the midline passing upwards into the neck and jaws and down the left arm into the fingers. The patient feels he is held in a vice and the intensity of the pain makes him sweat, while breathing may be difficult. There may be no warning of the event, though he may admit to previously experiencing the characteristic pain of angina pectoris. This is a similar but less severe discomfort that occurs during exertion, is relieved by rest and indicates disease of the coronary arteries.

By contrast, pain which comes from the lungs is a sharp, searing pain, localized to the area of disease. Breathing and coughing makes the pain worse and respirations are shallow and panting. This is the pain of pleurisy and results from involvement of the pleura following infection or infarction of lung tissue. With the former, known as pneumonia, there is infected sputum, green or yellow in appearance, and other symptoms associated with any febrile illness. Infarction of the lung is an occasional consequence of a pulmonary embolism, when a clot of blood in the venous circulation lodges in a branch of the pulmonary artery thereby starving the lung tissue beyond of its blood supply. Pain from the pericardium is similar to pleuritic pain but is related to posture, being relieved by sitting forward. It is produced by a pericarditis, of which there are several causes.

Pain may come from the dorsal spine or the rib cage – either the bones themselves, or the muscles attached to them. It is localized to the area of disease and often accompanied by local tenderness. Movement rather than exertion makes the pain worse but this may include movements of respiration making the distinction from pleuritic pain difficult in some cases. A history of chest injury is a useful clue.

Pain from the esophagus occurs with reflux of the stomach contents into the gullet. It is similar to heart pain, but is not related to exertion, is generally less severe, and is rapidly resolved by antacid mixtures or a glass of milk. The reflux tends to occur in the supine position and the patient is frequently troubled by pain at night. Rupture of the esophagus is much more dramatic. It is a rare complication of esophageal dilatation, the patient is profoundly shocked and death is common.

Clinical examination is important for patient assessment as well as for diagnostic purposes. Pulse, blood pressure, temperature and respiratory rate are recorded in all patients. In those with pericarditis or pleuritic pain the finding of a friction rub – a scratching noise related to respiratory movement heard with the stethoscope over the site of the pain – is useful for confirmation of the diagnosis. The jugular venous pressure may be raised in pulmonary embolism and following a myocardial infarction when there is evidence of heart failure as well. In the rare case of shingles presenting as chest pain, the typical vesicular rash may be seen in a nerve root distribution.

Useful investigations at this stage include an electrocardiograph (ECG, EKG) and X-rays of the chest, and when indicated, of ribs or dorsal spine. The X-rays would show pneumonia, lung infarction, rib fractures, dorsal spine disease, infiltration of lung or bone by tumour etc. The ECG would show the electrical aberrations associated with angina, myocardial infarction and pericarditis, together with abnormalities of heart rhythm.

MYOCARDIAL INFARCTION

If this is suspected either on the basis of history or with an atypical history but with suggestive ECG changes, the patient is normally transferred to a Coronary Care Unit.

The purpose of a Coronary Care Unit is to allow continuous observation and monitoring of the patient's heart during the first few days when serious and reversible disorders of rhythm are most likely to occur. Such rhythm disorders may also be witnessed in the Accident and Emergency department and it is important that the nurse should be familiar with some of them.

The most serious of all is a cardiac arrest in which the pumping action of the heart fails either from lack of electrical activity, asystole, when the ECG tracing is flat; or from uncoordinated ventricular muscle contractions, fibrillation, when the ECG is erratic and irregular and ventricular electrical complexes cannot be recognized. The patient collapses and stops breathing. The color drains from his face, blood pressure and peripheral and apical pulsations disappear. This is an absolute emergency for if normal circulation of oxygenated blood is not established within 3 minutes, irreversible brain damage will occur. Help must be summoned immediately by activating the Cardiac Arrest Team according to hospital custom. A sharp blow with the fist on the front of the patient's chest is always worthwhile and may be enough to restore an effective heart rhythm. If this is ineffective, however, the patient should be laid flat on his back on a firm surface such as the floor. Mouth-to-mouth resuscitation is begun at once with the neck held in extension, the jaws held forward and the patient's nose pinched between finger and thumb. A handkerchief between the resuscitator's and the patient's mouth makes the procedure acceptable, though it is preferable to use a Brook airway. Circulation of blood can be maintained by firm rhythmical pressure over the front of the chest with the palms of the hand, one placed on top of the other. This procedure, known as external cardiac massage, is better done by an assistant, and at a rate of 60 per minute. The ratio of massage to ventilation should be about 4 to 1, thus after every fourth massage, the assistant should pause to allow a single ventilation and so on. The Cardiac Arrest Team will usually include a doctor and an anesthetist as well as nursing personnel, porters and an ECG technician. Between them they will arrange the following:

(1) insertion of endotracheal tube and connection to a system of ventilation supplying oxygenated air (p. 222).
(2) insertion of intravenous line for sodium bicarbonate infusion and whatever drugs are considered necessary.
(3) connection to ECG monitor.

Meanwhile external cardiac massage must be continued. Once all this is achieved, everyone can relax a little for the immediate crisis is over. The doctor then decides, on the basis of the ECG tracing, the appropriate type of treatment to restore normal heart rhythm. For ventricular fibrillation, the commonest finding in this situation, a defibrillator is needed. This is a machine which gives a controlled electrical shock, which momentarily paralyzes the heart muscle, whereupon normal rhythm may return. Asystole may respond to an intracardiac injection of adrenaline (epinephrine).

Other heart rhythm abnormalities may be simply divided into fast ones (tachycardias) and slow ones (bradycardias), heart rates being in excess of 100 beats per minute with the former, and less than 50 beats per minute with the latter. A tachycardia may be either supraventricular or ventricular in type, depending upon the origin of the abnormality, and whether it is in the conducting system above the level of the ventricles or in the ventricular wall itself. This distinction is important when it comes to deciding the appropriate treatment and can be made on the appearance of the ECG. A supraventricular tachycardia can usually be controlled by drugs, whilst a ventricular tachycardia is better reversed, without delay, by electrical direct current (DC) cardioversion – a process similar in principle to defibrillation, in which the same machinery is used but after sedating the patient. A ventricular tachycardia often heralds fibrillation, hence the need for speed in treatment.

A bradycardia may result from slowing of the normal conducting system or from a block in conduction between the atria and ventricles. Treatment is not always necessary but the former, known as a sinus bradycardia, will respond to drugs, whilst the latter, known as atrioventricular dissociation will, if complete, require the insertion of an artificial pacemaker.

PLEURISY

A chest X-ray would indicate the cause of pleurisy in most cases. When it is due to pneumonia, the patient may occasionally be treated at home, but if a lung infarct is suspected, admission to the ward is necessary, so that anticoagulant treatment can begin. In both instances, adequate analgesics should be given, for this is a particularly unpleasant pain. Patients with pericarditis, a diagnosis made on clinical grounds and confirmed by ECG, are admitted to the general medical ward to determine its cause.

MUSCULO-SKELETAL PAIN

This can usually be controlled with anti-inflammatory and analgesic drugs and the patient allowed to return home.

ESOPHAGEAL PAIN

Antacids usually relieve the symptoms and 10 ml of magnesium trisilicate or aluminium hydroxide is worth trying. Abnormalities in the esophagus can be seen with the endoscope or indirectly by a barium swallow X-ray.

Upper gastrointestinal hemorrhage

Any patient who bleeds into the gastrointestinal tract must be admitted to hospital no matter how trivial the bleed might seem to be. The blood may appear in the vomit and be partly digested, appearing like coffee-grounds, or may be passed through the rectum when it is jet black in color and liquid in consistency, or both. The amount of blood loss is always difficult to estimate but is often more than appears at first sight. The reduction in circulatory blood volume, as occurs in a large hemorrhage from any source, produces sweating, pallor, faintness, a rapid heart rate and a fall in blood pressure – all the features of shock (p. 139). Thus the priority in management must be transfusion. The nurse is, therefore, expected to assist in resuscitation by preparing for an intravenous infusion. Blood is drawn for grouping and cross-matching and hemoglobin estimation. The intravenous line is kept open with normal saline unless it is judged that the patient is still bleeding when it will be necessary to infuse plasma until the matched blood is available. The principles of management are similar to those regarding hemorrhage from any source and have been described on page 135. The nurse's regular recordings of pulse and blood pressure, initially at no longer than 15 minute intervals, are invaluable as a guide to the rate of transfusion, and as an indication of continuing or recurrent hemorrhage. Thus the blood is run in at such a rate as to maintain a systolic blood pressure of 100 mmHg or more and a pulse rate of less than 100/min. A careful history and clinical examination at this stage can often indicate the cause and likely site of the bleeding, and the nurse should be aware of the more obvious possibilities. Drugs such as aspirin and the various non-steroidal anti-inflammatory agents, such as phenylbutazone, indomethacin, and ibuprofen may erode the lining of the stomach. Longstanding intermittent indigestion suggests a peptic ulcer. Blood appearing towards the end of prolonged vomiting from any cause is typical of an esophageal tear. A long history of alcohol abuse together with the various features of chronic liver disease such as jaundice, ascites, ankle swelling, spider naevi (a particular type of skin blemish) and splenic enlargement suggest the likelihood of esophageal varices. This last possibility is important to recognize for there are treatments in addition to transfusion which may be life-saving. Esophageal varices are distended veins in the wall of the esophagus which occur in disorders such as liver cirrhosis when there is obstruction to the flow of blood in the portal venous circulation. If one of these veins ruptures, bleeding may be torrential, especially as these patients will often have abnormal clotting as well. Surgical measures are required in the long term to control the bleeding and the medical staff will decide early on whether or not the patient is a candidate for surgery. However, as a temporary measure, the bleeding may stop in response to an intravenous injection of vasopressin – a drug which constricts blood vessels. Therefore, in any patient where bleeding esophageal varices is strongly suspected, immediate resuscitative measures must include 100 units of vasopressin in 100 ml given intravenously over 20 min. The nurse should be aware of the other consequences of treatment with vasopressin, for they indicate that an effective dose has been given:

colicky abdominal pain, sweating and defecation are amongst the more obvious.

Patients with gastrointestinal hemorrhage are quickly moved from the Accident and Emergency department to the general medical ward for investigation, which nowadays includes upper gastrointestinal endoscopy and surgical intervention if the bleeding does not stop of its own accord.

28

The breathless patient

M. B. McILLMURRAY

Patients presenting with breathlessness (dyspnea) in the Accident and Emergency department suffer a range of disorders requiring differing treatments and are a particular challenge to the skills of both nurses and doctors. Emergency treatment is often life-saving, whereas given inappropriately, it can be fatal. For example, high concentrations of oxygen are useful in severe pneumonias, but when given to patients whose only drive to respiration is the reduced level of oxygen in their blood it will cause breathing to cease (see p. 242). Similarly, sedative drugs which depress the respiratory drive are invaluable for patients with left ventricular failure, but dangerous in all forms of obstructive airways disease.

Whatever the cause of their breathlessness, patients are more comfortable sitting up and should be encouraged to do so. The nurse should remove the patient's clothing. Oxygen can be administered using a suitable mask (p. 244) such as a Ventimask but at concentrations no greater than 24% unless specifically prescribed by the doctor or if the condition is seen to rapidly deteriorate. The pulse, temperature, blood pressure and respiratory rate are recorded, and a calm and reassuring approach helps to allay the patient's anxiety. His color should be noted, as a deep blue color (cyanosis p. 162) is a grave sign. Other ominous signs include a systolic blood pressure of less than 100 mmHg, a pulse rate in excess of 100 and a cold and clammy periphery; if any of these are found, medical attention should be sought immediately.

The various causes of breathlessness can be considered as follows.

Disease of the lungs and air passages
OBSTRUCTION TO AIR FLOW
Simple mechanical obstruction to air flow may follow inhalation of a foreign body, external compression of the trachea or laryngeal edema and the treatment to remove or bypass the obstruction is self-evident.

Breathing demands a great deal of effort and may be accompanied by a loud high pitched sound, like the whistling of wind, known as stridor. The history is clearly important in indicating the diagnosis. When there is laryngeal obstruction an emergency tracheostomy may be necessary, though medical treatment should be sufficient in obstruction from oedema such as that in anaphylaxis (p. 295). Lung tumours, which compress the airways, present more insidiously and are treated with radiotherapy or cytotoxic chemotherapy.

Generalized airways obstruction, either from infection, inflammation and edema as in bronchitis, or from constriction of smooth muscle in the bronchial wall, as in asthma or both, is the commonest cause of breathlessness in the community. Acute bronchial infections are usually only life-threatening when they occur on a background of chronic bronchitis where patients may develop respiratory failure and die. A chronic productive cough and breathlessness with an abrupt worsening of symptoms in a cigarette smoker is the usual story. The sputum is purulent, the patient cyanosed and the breath-sounds inaudible because of the generalized wheeze. High concentrations of oxygen are dangerous (p. 242) for when the arterial blood CO_2 ($PaCO_2$) tension is high, the respiratory center in the brain is no longer sensitive to it, and the low arterial O_2 (PaO_2) level is the only way to drive the respiration; 24% oxygen (p. 243) can be given continuously and hydration, physiotherapy and antibiotics are the main components of treatment. Sedative drugs must not be used. The nurse should have a heparinized syringe (p. 236) and needle ready as arterial blood gas measurements will be urgently needed. Some patients may continue to deteriorate despite these measures. The rising $PaCO_2$ level causes confusion, drowsiness and coma. Swelling of the brain occurs and papilledema can be seen in the optic fundi. Respiratory stimulants such as doxapram, given by intravenous infusion, have been tried with some success but intermittent positive pressure ventilation must be considered at this stage (p. 221). However, this is inadvisable for patients who had been bed or chair bound by their disease in its chronic phase, for it is not possible to wean them from the machine. For the rest, however, mechanical ventilation offers a number of advantages such as reduction of dead space (p. 188) due to the presence of an endotracheal or tracheostomy tube, rest and sedation of the patient, and an efficient means of clearing the airways by suction. These patients are quickly transferred to the Intensive Care Unit.

The problems of patients with asthma are broadly similar. Sputum is notably absent, however, the obstruction being largely due to smooth muscle contraction. If the $PaCO_2$ is normal or reduced, then oxygen in concentrations of 28% or more can be used. Thus measurement of arterial blood gases is once more an essential part of management.

Asthma usually responds to bronchodilators and steroids, though large doses are often necessary. If mechanical ventilation is considered then the same conditions apply regarding patient selection. High inflation pressures are required to overcome the airways resistance.

ALVEOLAR DISEASE

Breathlessness may result from disorders of gas transfer; thus, the area of available alveolar tissue may be irreversibly diminished as in emphysema or temporarily reduced as in pneumonia. Moreover, diffusion of gas may be slowed by thickening of the alveolar wall as occurs in various disease states. Of these conditions, pneumonia is the one most likely to present acutely and thus appear in the Accident and Emergency department. The temperature is elevated, breathing may be rapid, shallow and painful. Fine crackling sounds (crepitations) can be heard over the involved parts of lung. High concentrations of oxygen can be safely used, antibiotics, physiotherapy and hydration are essential. A chest X-ray is helpful in confirming the diagnosis and determining the extent of the disease before transferring the patient to the general medical ward.

Diseases affecting the pleural cavity

Fluid or air may enter the intrapleural space and impede the function of the lungs. The degree of disability and breathlessness depends upon the size of the accumulation, its pressure on the underlying lung, and any associated lung disease. The one disorder presenting as a medical emergency is a steadily increasing accumulation of air in the pleural cavity, known as a tension pneumothorax. This arises from a small hole in the substance of one lung which allows air to pass from the lung into the pleural cavity during inspiration, but not in the reverse direction during expiration. The lung collapses and the pressure in that side of the chest steadily increases. The mediastinum is pushed towards the other side and the function of the other lung becomes impeded. The patient is normally fit and young and experiences a sharp pain when the pneumothorax first occurs. He then becomes increasingly breathless, ultimately cyanosed and dies if the pressure is not relieved. The trachea and heart apex can be felt to be displaced away from the affected side. The affected side is resonant, but silent to auscultation with the stethoscope. The nurse should prepare for the insertion of a chest drain, a flexible tube inserted anteriorly through the second intercostal space of the affected side. Air comes out under pressure with an immediate improvement in the patient's symptoms and appearance. The tube is then connected to an underwater seal. If the patient's condition is desperate it is justifiable to pass a 21 G needle through the chest wall until the drainage system can be prepared.

Diseases affecting blood circulation in the lungs

The lungs have a very rich blood supply and any major disturbance to blood flow will cause breathlessness. The pulmonary veins become distended if there is obstruction to the circulation in the left side of the heart, e.g. from narrowing of the mitral or aortic valves or from left ventricular failure. Pulmonary vascular distension stiffens the lungs and makes breathing more of an effort. Fluid may pass from the smallest blood vessels into the alveolar spaces giving rise to pulmonary edema and interfering with gas transfer. This process may develop insidiously and patients may complain of breathlessness only on exertion or when lying flat in bed at night. However, when left ventricular failure occurs abruptly the presentation is much more dramatic. The patient has a feeling of suffocation and is greatly distressed, agitated and frightened. Beads of sweat may appear on his forehead. If the left ventricular failure is the result of a heart attack, he will have chest pain as well. Medical attention must be sought immediately to prevent the patient from drowning in his own fluids.

Meanwhile, the nurse should stay with the patient who should be sat upright and breathing 40% oxygen through a Ventimask (p. 244). The pulse and blood pressure should be checked because left ventricular failure can result from either very slow or very fast abnormal heart rhythms, and from hypertension. The pulse should also be noted for its regularity since some of the more sinister heart rhythm disturbances are irregular. An ECG (EKG) will be recorded, but the medical priority is the relief of symptoms. The patient is normally given morphine or diamorphine, which will immediately relieve his distress. Both drugs cause nausea and vomiting and these side-effects are prevented by giving an anti-emetic at the same time. The potent diuretics such as frusemide (furosemide), given intravenously, produce a dramatic increase in urine flow and relieve the lung congestion. Any rhythm abnormality requires appropriate treatment and this may include electrical DC conversion as an emergency. A chest X-ray may be usefully arranged on the way from the Accident and Emergency department to the general medical ward.

Diseases affecting the muscles of respiration

Breathing is a complex procedure in which the ribs and muscles of the chest wall function like a bellows sucking and squeezing air in and out of the lungs during each respiratory cycle. Disease may affect these muscles or the nerves which control them, impair air intake and produce the sensation of air hunger and suffocation. Patients become restless and cyanosed. Thus chest wall movements are slight and breathing is shallow. Two of the more important disorders to recognize are myasthenia gravis, a muscle disease and polyneuropathy, a disease of nerves.

Myasthenia gravis is due to a disturbance in the conduction of impulses at the interface between nerve and muscle. The characteristic clinical feature is an abnormal fatiguability of muscles, and in most cases the earliest to be involved are those supplied by the cranial nerves. Double vision and weakness of swallowing and chewing are common symptoms, hence it is unusual for myasthenia gravis to present with breathlessness. Any muscle may be involved, however, and in severe examples, respiratory failure may develop. The diagnosis will likely be known if the patient comes to the Accident and Emergency department as a medical emergency. Fortunately, the disease responds dramatically to anticholinesterase drugs, such as neostigmine and pyridostigmine. A short-acting preparation, edrophonium, can be given intravenously with immediate and dramatic results. This is a useful diagnostic test. There is one note of caution. Patients with myasthenia gravis receiving too large a dose of an anticholinesterase will deteriorate and the respiratory muscles may become paralyzed. The treatment of this crisis is intermittent positive pressure ventilation and a cholinesterase reactivator, such as pralidoxime, given in frequent small doses. Failure to respond to edrophonium in a myasthenic indicates this possibility.

A polyneuropathy is a rare sequel to a virus infection (Guillain-Barré syndrome). The damaged peripheral nerves initially affect the hands and feet and numbness and paresthesiae are amongst the earliest symptoms. The process slowly spreads proximally to a varying degree, but the nerves supplying the respiratory muscles can be involved. The reflexes in the affected limbs are lost, there is muscle weakness and sensory loss. Mechanical ventilation may be required and large doses of steroids are usually given. Fortunately, the majority eventually recover completely.

29

The child patient

A. H. DAVIES

Some hospitals reserve special waiting, examination and treatment areas in the Accident and Emergency department for the child patient. They are usually brightly decorated with pictures and posters on the walls and are well supplied with plenty of toys and play apparatus. These provide the child with a more familiar and understandable environment and help to allay the bewilderment and fear which arise from injury and pain. Another advantage is that the worried child is not made worse by the impersonal atmosphere of a large busy general Accident and Emergency department, with its bandaged and bleeding people, crutches and wheelchairs, and uniformed nurses hurrying about their duties.

The adult patient benefits too, because he is spared the ordeal of seeing and listening to the cries and shrieks of frightened children. Also it is much more pleasant for the nursing staff to treat a child who is calm, quiet and cooperative.

Unfortunately, most children have to attend traditional departments. Nevertheless, some steps can be taken to welcome the child and make him feel more at home and to calm his fears.
For example:

(1) Wherever possible the small child should be given priority and not kept waiting longer than is absolutely necessary. Most adults are very understanding and do not object to a child 'jumping the queue', particularly if it is very noisy.

(2) A cupboard or large box should be supplied with a selection of soft toys, wooden animals and simple games which can be brought out for the child to play with or hold. The child should also be allowed to keep its own favourite toy, or little blanket comforter which many children cherish.

(3) The waiting room can be partly child-orientated with some of the posters selected to interest children rather than adults. A large tankful of tropical fish is well known to soothe and

fascinate child and adult alike. Usually the proprietor of the local tropical fish store will agree to keep a tank stocked and cleaned, sometimes free of charge, in exchange for its advertising value.

(4) It is most important to talk to the child patient, and not confine question and conversation to the accompanying adult. If the nurse asks the child what happened, and sympathizes with him, discusses the situation and explains what is going to happen, she makes the child feel important and interesting and is often successful in gaining his cooperation, so that management and treatment are easier.

(5) Although masks are usually worn when examining and treating open wounds and burns in the adult patient, they should be discarded when dealing with children except in the presence of deep wounds and large areas of burn.

(6) Parents should normally be encouraged to stay with the child during treatment. In the past parents were asked to wait outside the treatment area, partly because some children behave better without their parents, and also because of the theory that parents should not be associated with a painful and unpleasant procedure. However, it is now felt that children should not be made to feel abandoned by their parents. Also, the parents themselves may feel happier if allowed to watch and be reassured that the infant is being handled sensibly and treated with gentleness and care. Nevertheless, some parents are squeamish and do not care to watch: therefore, every case must be considered on its own merit. The parent is given the choice, and if he decides to remain he can be made to feel useful by holding the child's hands or head.

(7) The use of sedation, analgesia and local or general anesthesia should be considered more frequently with the child than the adult, to ensure that memory of the occasion is less unpleasant should he have to attend again. Furthermore, any procedure needing time and care, such as suturing a facial laceration, is easier and more likely to produce a satisfactory result in the absence of struggling and restraint in a frightened child.

The screaming child

It has been already stated that many children cry and make a fuss when they are brought to hospital because they are frightened of the injury and the strangeness of the surroundings. However, it must be remembered that crying may be partly or entirely due to pain, and will never be alleviated by the patience and sensible handling described above. For example, a screaming burned or scalded toddler or infant should be brought straight through to the treatment area, without waiting for the formalities of registration and documentation, and the doctor summoned to prescribe an intravenous or intramuscular analgesic such as morphia. The dosage chart should be readily available, possibly on the inside door of the poisons cupboard, so that it is not mislaid and the appropriate dosage for age and size of the child can be instantly checked. An estimation of weight is necessary because in the emotional trauma of the event the average mother may not remember the child's weight, and the average father may never have known!

Poisoning in children

Although adult poisoning is dealt with in Chapter 11 some particulars of the treatment of poisoned children merit special attention.

All children as they grow and develop constantly learn about the world around them, testing their surroundings with their various senses. One of the easiest ways of discovering the nature of an object or substance is to put it in the mouth, to taste and feel it with the lips and tongue, perhaps with disastrous results.

The majority of potentially poisoned children brought to the department are between the ages of 18 months and 3 years: there are often predisposing factors at home. For example:

(1)   Someone in the home may be ill, so that tablets and medicines are left lying around. The child himself may have been ill and knows he pleases his mother by taking his medicine.
(2)   Recent illness, bereavement or domestic problems may cause the mother to relax her normal vigilance and care of the child.
(3)   There may be a lack of understanding by the mother of the curious and exploratory nature of her developing child, so that cupboards are inadequately fastened and medicines and tablets not kept in a locked medicine cabinet.
(4)   Grandma or other sick elderly relatives may visit the home and leave a handbag containing tablets on the floor or low table.
(5)   The child may visit friends or relatives who have no small children and are not in the habit of child-proofing their cupboards.

SUBSTANCES TAKEN

Children are brought into the Accident and Emergency department having taken an endless variety of poisons. The author has treated poisoned children who have ingested such diverse substances as:

Nail polish	Rat poison	Contraceptives
Bleach	Firelighters	Toilet deodorizer blocks
Disinfectant	Analgesics	Cat worming tablets
Hair dye	'Heart' tablets	Wood preservative
Turpentine	Tranquillizers	Whisky, gin, sherry etc.
Weed killer	Liquid detergents	

Action
It must be decided:

(1) What substance has been taken?
(2) Is it really poisonous?
(3) How much has been taken?

IDENTIFICATION
During the last few years many advances have been made to protect the public. For example, most medicine bottles are now labelled with the name of their contents, and dangerous agents are usually labelled 'poison'. Many manufacturers market their products in 'child-proof' containers but those are not infallible because many bright children, given sufficient time, find the secret of opening even these containers.

Any substance in an unlabelled bottle must be considered poisonous and treatment started (see below) while an attempt is made to establish its identification. Sometimes its appearance or smell help identification and the biochemical laboratory may help, but the expense of a full chemical analysis will probably not be undertaken merely on suspicion that the child has taken some potential poison or before some signs of poisoning appear.

Whilst enquiries and decisions are being made, the child should be undressed and examined, the pulse, respiration and temperature recorded and particular note taken of any evidence of spilled substances on the child's hands, clothing, lips or in the mouth.

After identification of the ingested substance, if doubt exists about its toxic effects or the method of treatment, advice is obtainable at the poison centres, usually situated in teaching hospitals, such as Guy's Hospital London, Edinburgh Royal Infirmary, and Leeds Infirmary. Their telephone numbers should be readily available in every Emergency department.

TREATMENT
Decision is made as to whether the substances taken should be eliminated, and if so what method to use.

In general, caustic or volatile substances should not be eliminated because when swallowed they burn the mouth, pharynx, esophagus and stomach, so that if they are vomited back their effect is doubled. Furthermore, any attempt to wash them out by passing a stomach tube may further damage the esophagus and possibly perforate its wall.

Volatile substances such as petrol (gasoline) mainly damage the lungs and may be inhaled during vomiting irrespective of whether it is induced by a stomach tube or emetic.

Most tablets and medicines are taken in relatively small quantities and vomiting is induced by giving an emetic such as 15–30 ml tincture of ipecacuanha. It is given to the child by either the nurse or the parent, and when safely swallowed is followed by a cupful of whatever drink the child may be induced to take, such as milk, water, or a 'fizzy' favourite. The child is then left with the parents and a vomit bowel, a story book and a good supply of paper towels. The author has never known ipecacuanha to fail, though it may be 15–20 minutes before vomiting begins.

STOMACH WASHOUT IN CHILDREN
Substances such as iron tablets, paraquat and other weed killers must be eliminated quickly and completely by stomach tube. It is inadvisable to wait for an emetic to take effect. Iron compounds are the commonest cause of death from poisoning in children.

Specific treatment consists of aspirating the iron through a stomach tube and introducing down the tube as quickly as possible the unpleasant tasting iron chelating agent desferrioxamine. This causes the soluble iron salt to precipitate out of solution into a non-soluble substance so preventing its absorption into the blood stream.

Desferrioxamine must also be given intramuscularly. Dosage of both forms of desferrioxamine depends on the weight of the patient.

Nursing management of stomach washout

(1) The parents are sent for a walk or directed to an area as far away from the child as possible, since this is one situation where they may become so disturbed and distressed at the unpleasantness of the procedure that they may interfere with its progress.

(2) The child is undressed down to its underpants and its shoes are always removed, since a well aimed kick can be very uncomfortable and disconcerting.

(3) The child is wrapped firmly and securely in a cotton blanket or sheet, round his whole body, legs and arms, leaving only his head exposed (see Figure 10.2).

(4) The child is placed on his side on a trolley (gurney), with his head right up to the top end of the trolley which is tilted slightly head down.

(5) At least three nurses or helpers are essential. One holds the

wrapped child from her position at the side of the trolley, the one at the head end introduces and keeps the tube in the child's mouth and stomach and prevents it from slipping out, and the third uses the jug and funnel.

(6) *Necessary apparatus*
   (a) Warm water (5–10 l)
   (b) A large bore rubber stomach tube lubricated with jelly. An adult who takes an overdose is miserable and depressed and is unlikely to have eaten a hearty meal. A child, however, is likely to have eaten breakfast or lunch and his stomach may be full of incompletely chewed food which will not return via a small bore tube. He therefore requires the largest bore tube that can be passed.
   (c) A large funnel and jug.
   (d) A clear 2 gallon bucket to collect the washed-out fluid.
   (e) Plastic apron and floor covering – a little vomit goes a long way.

(7) *Method.* If possible the child is persuaded to open his mouth so that the tube can be introduced. Tact and persuasion may work, but sometimes the tube must be popped in quickly when the child opens his mouth to cry, or when the nostrils are deliberately blocked by the nurse's fingers thus making him open his mouth to breathe.

The tube must be passed quickly and firmly down to a pre-positioned 'average toddler' mark which however is adjusted for a larger or smaller child. Although the gastric tube is fairly comfortable when *in situ*, it usually provokes vomiting during its insertion, so the nurse must be ready to avoid being covered by the gastric contents and catch them in a suitable receiver. The funnel is filled with water from the jug and then elevated to allow gravity to nearly empty the funnel of its water down the tube into the child's stomach. The funnel is then lowered and the stomach contents are syphoned into the bucket. This procedure must be repeated until the washings are clear. If the child bites the tube and impedes the flow of fluid, the nurse should not attempt to prise open the jaws or the child will bite her fingers. Usually the child relaxes his bite after a few minutes but if he fails to do so the nostrils are again occluded between the nurse's finger and thumb.

(8) When the washings are sufficiently clear the tube is quickly removed and the child is allowed to sit up. He is cleaned and dried, then cuddled and made a fuss of while being dressed, and told what a good child he has been. The parents are then allowed to return.

Nurses involved in the washout of a child's stomach always find the procedure distressing and physically and emotionally exhausting, and consequently are usually very careful to keep drugs and poisons out of reach of their own children.

Further management
Whether or not the child is allowed home depends upon the decision of the doctor and the commonsense of the parents.

It is at this point that the nurse may be able to offer some advice about the safe storage of medicines, tablets and poisonous household substances. At the same time, trying to maintain a non-censorius attitude, she may also be able to deliver a few hints about child care and management.

Some Accident and Emergency departments have liaison arrangements with community health visiting nurses who may follow up an 'overdose' attendance with a home visit.

30

Non-accidental injury to children

A. H. DAVIES

Non-accidental injury to children (NAI) refers to their ill-treatment by parents or guardians, and embraces physical or mental neglect or actual physical injury. NAI has now replaced the term 'Battered Baby Syndrome' because children older than babies are involved and besides being battered they may be shaken, burned or deliberately poisoned, and to avoid the emotive impact of the term.

History of cruelty to children
Throughout the ages people have deliberately inflicted physical harm and injury on others weaker and more vulnerable than themselves. Most children cannot defend themselves against adults and many children have perished over the centuries at the hands of their parents. Harsh treatment and infanticide are still regarded with varying degrees of tolerance in different countries and in some primitive societies female children are still considered to be disposable.

In the mid-19th century with the growth of cities and industrial civilization the number of children surviving birth and infancy began to increase, and with overcrowding and poverty many families were unable to adequately cope with them. Conversely, about the same time, public awareness and concern began to grow regarding poverty, misery and deprivation and a 'humanitarian' movement appeared among writers and politicians. One problem which many of them considered with increasing concern was the inhuman way in which children were beaten, starved, and employed for long hours in dreadful conditions. Dickens wrote about cruelty in many of his novels and Lewis Carroll mentioned it in *Alice in Wonderland*. Alice was worried about the way the Duchess treated her baby and heard her singing:

> Speak roughly to your little boy,
> and beat him when he sneezes,
> He only does it to annoy
> Because he knows it teases.

Meanwhile the baby was being shaken and Alice felt that if it were not removed the Duchess would surely kill it.

When attempts were made to protect children from the harsh treatment of their parents considerable opposition was encountered. Children were considered to be the possessions of their parents, and so had no individual rights. There was no law to protect them until the latter part of the 19th century when the first prosecutions for cruelty to children were made in Great Britain and North America, under laws concerning cruelty to animals.

In the early 1950s an American orthopedic surgeon called Caffey described a number of babies who presented with bruising and multiple fractures in various stages of healing, and sometimes with retinal hemorrhage and brain damage, but with no history of injury. It became known as 'Caffey's syndrome' until it was realized that no history of injury was admitted because it was the parents themselves who had caused the injuries by beating, twisting and shaking their infants.

This then was the beginning of recognition of the 'Battered Baby Syndrome' and of the fact that tiny babies could be ill-treated as well as older children, and that it was not necessarily a 'disease' of poverty.

DETECTION

It is obviously important to be aware of the possibility of NAI and to detect minor injuries before the child has been seriously injured and his life endangered. The main basis of detection is communication between all people who have contact with children, whenever any suspicion of trouble is aroused. So, suspicion of NAI must never be suppressed; on the contrary it should be communicated to responsible authorities as soon as possible.

Obviously the staff in an Accident and Emergency department are in a good position to recognize child abuse in its early stages, when only minor injuries are present, and certainly must be aware of the action to take when more definite serious injuries occur.

Consequently the nurse should recognize the factors which help her to suspect and detect that all is not well. These are:

(1) *History* of the cause of the injury should be compatible with the actual injury present. For example, it is unusual for a child to trip over and fracture his femur – he is more likely to have fallen from at least his own height or have had his leg deliberately bent or twisted. Scalding of the buttocks is unlikely to occur if a child has pulled a kettle of hot water on himself, and a fall down stairs rarely produces bruising at the back of the knees.

(2) *Absence* of history when there is an obvious and fairly serious fracture such as that of the femur or skull.

(3) *Delay* between injury and attendance. The usual and natural reaction of parents to an accidental injury in their child is to seek medical advice fairly soon – usually within 1–2 hours of its occurrence.

(4) *The child*, if old enough to realize what is happening may be too frightened to talk about the injury, although occasionally a toddler will be very frank when the parent is absent and say 'Daddy hit me' or 'Mummy bit me' or 'She pushed me downstairs'. The child may be quiet and withdrawn and not appear to relate well to his parents. He may duck or hide his face when approached by the nurse or doctor. Occasionally, a small child may have an expression of frozen awareness, as if always waiting for something awful to happen.

Sometimes the converse is true and the child who is perpetually ill treated by his parents may be abnormally and indiscriminately friendly and cooperative with strangers.

The child may be small for his age, undernourished, dirty, cold, ill clad and look generally uncared for. In spite of the fact that the problem of NIA can occur in all social strata, there are, nevertheless, a majority of known 'at risk' children living in poor social conditions associated with unemployment, bad housing, one parent families, drink problems and general inadequacies.

(5) *The parents* may be young and seem immature or withdrawn and uncommunicative, and even unconcerned about their child. Sometimes, however, they are effusive, calling the child 'darling' all the time, while giving the impression they have never used the term before, often repeating again and again that they cannot think how the injury happened. Others may handle the child or children roughly and unsympathetically.

(6) *Repeated visits* by the child to the Accident and Emergency department for injuries which appear trivial, may be an attempt to allay the neighbours' suspicions or because of the fear that for once they may have gone too far and really caused damage. Occasionally, however, bringing a deliberately injured child to hospital may be a way of seeking attention for the problem – a sort of 'cry for help'.

(7) *Variations in history* may be given even by the same person to the receptionist, nurse, doctor, radiographer etc. It is therefore always worthwhile for everyone who has to deal with an injured child to ask 'What happened?' or 'How did you do it?'

(8) *The injuries* a child has received can, to the 'practised eye' arouse suspicions to the possibility of parental abuse.

Once a child is mobile he is liable to accidental injury under

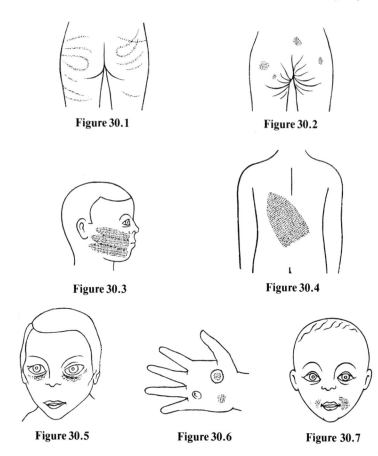

Figure 30.1   Figure 30.2

Figure 30.3   Figure 30.4

Figure 30.5   Figure 30.6   Figure 30.7

Figure 30.1–7   Injuries probably of non-accidental origin

Figure 30.1   Bruises on buttocks caused by a strap or belt
Figure 30.2   Signs of neglect and injury – wasting of buttocks and discrete bruises which are unlikely to be due to accidental injury
Figure 30.3   Finger slap bruising
Figure 30.4   Burn with a recognizable shape – unlikely to be caused by accident
Figure 30.5   Bilateral 'black eyes' – and face with anxious expression
Figure 30.6   Small discrete burns on palm – different stages of healing – probably due to cigarette burns
Figure 30.7   Bruising of soft tissues around mouth, unlikely to be due to an accident. May be inflicted when trying to force a small child or baby to take food

the care of the most conscientious and caring parents. However, the pattern of accidental injuries is fairly standard. A small child usually falls forwards and takes his weight on the hands and elbows, and bangs his forehead, knees and shins. If the bruising does not conform with this 'normal' pattern, special note should be made of where the bruising is. Bruises around the neck or on the cheeks, the front of the abdomen or the chest, the backs of the knees and flexor aspects of the arms should immediately arouse suspicion. Other minor injuries which suggest abuse, are bruises and burns with a recognizable pattern that have been made with a definite object, such as a strap, stick, cigarette end, or an iron (Figures 30.1–30.7). Human bite marks are very characteristic and recognizable, as are hand-slap marks or finger tip bruises especially on the face or around the child's waist or chest due to being roughly lifted up and shaken.

In addition to new bruising of suspicious character there may be other bruises present, of various colors, ranging from the most recent to red, blue, black, green and eventually yellow, indicating that the child may have been repeatedly abused and not just injured in an isolated loss of parental control.

ACTION

It is inadvisable for the nurse and doctor who first see and examine an injured child to disclose their suspicions to the accompanying parent, or to accuse them of causing a deliberate injury. They immediately become annoyed and may remove the child without treatment, and not return for further treatment or bring the child with any new injury.

The nurse should not adopt a disapproving attitude because at times all children are illogical and unreasonable. Anyone in charge of them may be worn out by their constant crying, and be exasperated by their irrational and stubborn behaviour, particularly if associated with unfavourable social conditions. In these circumstances the person's self-control may snap – 'There but for the grace of God go I' is a wise maxim.

It is rare for an individual, or even the combined members of one department to be able to make the definite decision that an injury is non-accidental, or that a child is undoubtedly being injured by its parents.

Usually the suspicious factors are insufficient for them to be sure that the case is one involving child abuse. Therefore, any minor suspicion should be brought to the attention of the social services and a case conference arranged, embracing representatives from any discipline which might know the child, such as his school, hospital, probation service or community health service etc. Then the whole circumstances of the child and his family can be discussed and a corporate opinion be formed as to whether the child is really 'at risk' from non-accidental injury.

It must be emphasized that all knowledge or suspicions must be treated as very confidential and should *never* be discussed with anyone not concerned with the case.

31

The elderly patient

A. H. DAVIES

Although the average age of the population of the western world is gradually increasing, families are becoming more unwilling to take responsibility for the care and supervision of the welfare of elderly relatives. They utter all kinds of reasons and excuses, some valid and some rather doubtful, such as 'We have no room' or 'We are both out at work all day' or 'It would disturb the children'. Sometimes they claim to have a bad back or a bad heart or that their doctor has advised against them taking on further responsibility. Many elderly people have no relatives and either live alone in unsatisfactory conditions or rely on old peoples' homes, sheltered accommodation and geriatric wards, all of which are full and have long waiting lists. These problems must always be anticipated and considered when an elderly patient is brought to the Accident and Emergency department.

Collapse

The nurse should lay the elderly collapsed patient on a couch or trolley (gurney) and make a quick assessment of his general appearance. If he is breathless, in pain, shocked, or unconscious, she must send for the doctor immediately either by using the emergency call system or with the help of another person; she should not leave the patient unattended. This type of patient is then dealt with in exactly the same way as those in a younger age group. However, many elderly people are brought to hospital in reasonably good general condition having collapsed whilst shopping, visiting friends, attending social clubs or church. They may have some minor illness or be overtired having tried to do too much, or may have missed a meal and become faint.

The nurse can do much to reassure the patient and make him comfortable until the cause of the collapse is diagnosed.

Her duties include:

(1) Talking to the patient concerning what happened and

corroborating the history with the ambulance man, relative or friend present at the time the accident occurred.

(2) Maintaining a flow of 'small talk' whilst counting the pulse and respiratory rates and measuring the blood pressure. Provided that these are reasonably normal she can sit the patient up; few elderly patients like to lie flat.

(3) Finding out whether the patient has wet or soiled clothes and asking whether he or she needs a bedpan or bottle.

(4) Ensuring that the patient is comfortable and fit enough to provide the administrator with details of name, address, next of kin etc.

(5) Explaining that the doctor will come along, examine him, find out what caused the incident and decide if he is fit to go home.

(6) Undressing the patient for examination. This may be difficult because old people often wear many layers of clothing and may need gentle persuasion to remove them. When undressed the patient must be provided with a hospital gown or temporary garments because the elderly feel very insecure covered by only one or two thin blankets, and even though it is probably very warm inside the hospital they are often used to heavy bed-clothes and will complain of feeling cold.

The nurse must try to appreciate that admission procedures upset and confuse elderly patients, some of whom have never been inside a hospital before and have many unspoken fears and worries. The nurse should maintain frequent contact with the elderly patient particularly when he has to wait a long time for examination and treatment, or for ambulance transport to take him home, so that he does not feel alone, forgotten or neglected. He may need reminding why he is there, even where he is and what he is waiting for, and a little general conversation will help reassure him that he is among friends. The nurse should offer food and drink provided they are permitted by the doctor and again ask about the need for a bedpan or urine bottle. If the patient has to wait for more than an hour or so he should be encouraged to change position regularly, with help if needed, particularly if he is large and immobile, to avoid numbness and the possible formation of pressure sores. If the patient has been examined, treated and is waiting to go home he will be happier if he is dressed again and usually prefers to sit in a chair rather than lie on an examination couch or trolley.

FALLS
Physical injuries are common in elderly people. The sense of balance diminishes with age and a minor trip or stumble, which in youth is quickly righted, becomes a heavy fall in the elderly, particularly if the

person is obese. In addition, he often finds it very difficult or impossible to get up again causing considerable emotional and sometimes physical upset.

Common injuries in the elderly are:

Face and scalp lacerations and hematomata
Colles' fractures
Fractures of the neck of the humerus and sometimes dislocation of the shoulder
Fractures of the ribs
Crush fractures of lumbar vertebrae
Ankle sprains and fractures
Fractures of the neck of the femur

In the elderly, minor falls may produce major fractures, due to osteoporosis which increases with age, particularly in women. The ease with which elderly bones break causes an anomaly in priorities when treating elderly patients with fractures. Pain is not such a prominent complaint in the elderly, but distress is very marked, caused by the upset of the incident and worry about its possible consequences. The nurse may have to expend time and patience in reassurance and repeated explanation of what is likely to happen and less time in achieving pain relief.

Occasionally, however, this apparent lack of pain associated with a fairly major injury is due to the greater degree of stoicism that old people show towards pain. Many of them were brought up in a time when children were taught to 'grin and bear' pain and not to complain. Also many old people suffer chronic pain all the time, so that a new pain neither surprises nor upsets them so much.

It is, therefore, wise to enquire whether there are any other pains and bruises elsewhere and to undress the patient sufficiently to enable the doctor to make a full examination.

The author once had a very embarrassing experience when treating an old lady for a Colles' fracture. She had been attending hospital for about 6 weeks, always sitting in a wheelchair. This was not surprising in itself because in busy clinics elderly and frail people are sometimes put in a wheelchair for speed and ease of movement. Eventually she was asked if she needed the chair, whereupon the patient admitted that she had been unable to walk since the fall that had produced the wrist fracture, but she had not considered it sufficiently important to mention. After X-ray examination had disclosed a fractured neck of femur the author had the task of explaining to the relatives that the patient had to be admitted to hospital for an operation.

To the elderly living alone even a minor injury or illness becomes a major problem. They are unable to cope and may even require admission to a hospital for a condition that does not justify the involvement of the acute nursing and medical services. These social admissions can be a burden to orthopaedic surgeons and nursing staff because once the elderly person is institutionalized, even for only a few days, he suddenly becomes very dependent and may become confused and disorientated, and then cannot be sent home.

After treating an old person in the Accident and Emergency department the nurse has several further duties to perform:

(1) Arrange for follow-up and after care by the general practitioner or in the hospital out-patient department.

(2) Arrange suitable transport for the patient's return to hospital and ensure he understands the date and time of day it will call to collect him from home.

(3) Instruct the patient about the care of any injury, e.g. whether rest or exercise is advisable.

The nurse should given written instructions concerning the above advice and arrangements, but should realize that they may be lost or forgotten in the depths of a pocket or handbag and never looked at again. Therefore, she should also issue verbal instructions and repeat them several times to the patient and to any available relative or friend.

(4) The nurse must see the elderly person stand and walk unaided if he is being sent home alone. A walking stick or walking frame may help but they are of little use if he also needs the additional support of another person. It is unrealistic to expect any elderly person to cope with crutches and avoid weight bearing on a newly plastered leg, if the material used is the ordinary plaster of Paris (p. 66). However, some of the newer synthetic cast materials such as 'Baycast' 'Scotchcast' or 'Hexolite' are sometimes preferred, because they dry more quickly and permit weight bearing before the patient leaves the department. They are too expensive to use for every patient but their cost may be justified if it saves the old person from being admitted to hospital.

(5) The nurse should arrange care at the patient's home while he is partly incapacitated. She can contact friends and relatives or a community nurse to visit with dressings or toilet and ask the social welfare department to arrange a home help.

Sometimes family doctors send elderly patients to hospital after a minor fall, hoping that at last places will be found for them in a geriatric unit or old peoples' home. However, some geriatricians insist that patients are not accepted directly from the Accident and Emergency department. Although this may appear harsh it does save the department from becoming a convenient dumping ground for unwanted old folk.

Finally, throughout the nurse's dealings with old people she must remember that however deaf, confused, dirty, demanding or difficult they may be, they are still human beings and she must treat them with courtesy, consideration and respect and a great deal of kindness.

32

The violent patient

A. H. DAVIES

More and more departments, particularly in big cities, are experiencing bouts of violence within their premises, resulting in injury to hospital staff and property. The nurse must know why violence occurs, how to protect herself and prevent the patient from hurting himself.

Violence and illness

Violent behaviour may be a manifestation of the following conditions:

(1) Head injury
(2) Cerebrovascular accident
(3) Epilepsy (and pseudo-epilepsy or hysteria)
(4) Confusion in elderly patients
(5) Hypoglycemia
(6) Overdose of drugs
(7) Withdrawal effect in drug addicts
(8) Acute alcoholic intoxication
(9) Alcohol deprivation (withdrawal effect, delirium tremens)
(10) Mental subnormality
(11) Psychiatric illness such as schizophrenia or manic-depression.

Any attempt to undress, examine or treat a patient sometimes provokes alarming reactions in the above conditions.

The violent behaviour of the psychotic may be triggered off by a tactless word or even by a nurse's manner or accent. Minor arguments about the competence of the doctor or racial considerations can sometimes flare into full scale abuse and eventually violence.

PREVENTION OF VIOLENCE AND DEALING WITH THE PATIENT

(1) The nurse should anticipate the possibility of a restless and irritable patient becoming violent. All patients who are

conscious should be treated with tact and courtesy even if they do not appear to be fully aware of what is going on; a tone of condescension or disapproval may penetrate a confused mind and produce an undesirable reaction.

(2) The nurse should not start or continue to undress a belligerent patient for examination, or attempt to treat him if he decides to resist. Furthermore, she must not become annoyed and abusive herself, but should stop, send for help and attempt nothing further until the situation subsides.

(3) The nursing staff should not fight with a restless patient or attempt to hold him down, unless it is for the patient's protection. It is most unwise to try and administer drugs by injection without the patient's cooperation.

DEALING WITH RELATIVES AND FRIENDS
Every attempt should be made to avoid confrontations and arguments with complaining relatives or friends. An explanation of the situation and the provision of information before complaints are anticipated is the best way of preventing problems arising (p. 9).

Action
If despite her tact and patience and deliberate avoidance of confront-ation, a situation develops in which the nurse cannot prevent violence erupting, there are some general rules which the nurse should observe. However, every violent situation presents its own difficulties and needs handling in an individual way.

(1) No violent situation should be handled *alone*, the nurse must send for help immediately. All areas of the Accident and Emergency department should have an intercommunication system, involving alarm bells, buzzers or microphones. In hospitals where violence is common an agreed alarm call on the internal telephone should be devised, similar to the cardiac arrest call – for example using easily remembered numbers like 333 or 999. Official help can then be despatched immediately to the department, perhaps in the form of an 'incident team' including a male nurse, a senior female nurse and a porter.

(2) Damage to property should be ignored in an emergency situation – damage to persons is much more important.

(3) Opinions vary as how the nurse can best avoid personal injury. She has the choice of two techniques:
(a)   She should keep close in to the violent person – it is more difficult to hit or kick someone if he is very near.
(b)   She should keep well away from him so she is out of range.

Obviously every situation differs and in fact there may be no choice.

(4)   If the nurse decides to intervene when someone else is being attacked, she should approach from the rear, and grab the attacker round his chest forcing his elbows into his sides. An alternative is to grab his coat collar, pull his coat half way down his back, just off his shoulders, so that his arm movements are restricted.

Occasionally a violent person can be brought down by grabbing him around the knees from behind.

(5)   The nurse should never turn her back to a person threatening violence or she may be unprepared for the attack. What is more, the person may regard her turned back as an additional insult.

(6)   The nurse should contact the police. Their presence can be most re-assuring and helpful, and their very arrival may cause the situation to just 'melt away'. This may be a little embarrassing for the nurse who has called them, and makes her feel she has 'cried wolf' – but it is better than having a fight on her hands.

Some city Accident and Emergency departments have a direct link with the local police station. Such a facility should be requested if violent incidents in the department are becoming more frequent.

(7)   The nurse should ask for help from any doctors or other patients in the department – very few will refuse.

(8)   Any injuries sustained by the nurse or other staff or patients must receive prompt attention and treatment as soon as the incident is over. Details are entered into the hospital accident report book.

(9)   The incident should be fully recorded in writing as soon as possible while the sequence of events is still clear in the nurse's mind. Later the situation and its handling can be discussed by all staff involved, so that lessons may be learned for the future.

33

Hospital hoppers and the dead patient

A. H. DAVIES

Hospital hoppers

Some patients abuse the services of the hospital for their own purposes. They may present with very authentic symptoms of serious injury or illness, in order to gain admission or acquire strong narcotic drugs.

The commonest presenting complaint in these 'phoney' patients is chest pain which is usually graphically and accurately described. Another common symptom is loin pain simulating ureteric colic. Both pains merit the administration of diamorphine (heroin), morphia or pethidine (meperidine), if the symptoms are authentic enough to convince the doctor, because neither a myocardial infarction nor a ureteric stone can be conclusively disproved on first examination of the patient. Probably patients who use these, or any other, simulated symptoms have actually experienced the real thing in the past and may even be able to exhibit an abnormal ECG (EKG) or produce some blood-stained urine by artefact, to substantiate their story.

SUSPICIOUS FACTORS
The nurse may note:

(1) An over-plausible story
(2) Familiarity with hospital procedures
(3) A distant address
(4) That sometimes no 'next of kin' is reported
(5) Lack of concern that relatives or friends should be informed of his admission
(6) On undressing the patient for examination, puncture marks on the forearms, thighs or buttocks from previous injections, and abdominal scars from laparotomies
(7) The patient is vague about which hospitals he has attended before, or who is his usual general practitioner. On checking with the hospitals which he names, the nurse will find no record

of his attendance there, or else a story of similar incident followed by his sudden disappearance will be disclosed. His general practitioner may have a non-existent address.

Once suspicion is aroused the nurse consults the departmental files comprising a description, circulated by other hospitals, of similar patients after they have been tricked by the patient's act. In the author's hospital this is known as the 'Rogues' Gallery', but it should be realized that the patient may have several aliases and the name he gives may not correspond with the one used in the file.

ACTION

If the nurse or the doctor tells such a patient that there is some doubt about his authenticity, the patient often produces a great deal of verbal abuse, and may take fright and disappear. Cases of deception must be reported to the administrator and if any narcotics or dangerous drugs have been used the police should also be informed. The administrator then circulates other hospitals in the area with details of name, age, appearances and complaint, for entry into their own Rogues' Gallery.

The author remembers an interesting, if unusual, hospital hopper who once came to the Lancaster Accident and Emergency department. He was a male, aged 30 years, who walked in accompanied and supported by a 'friend'. He gave a history, corroborated by the friend, of working on a building site, falling from scaffolding about 20 feet from the ground, and grabbing at a horizontal pole to save himself, sustained a traction injury to the left arm. He complained of headache, stiff neck, paresthesiae and pain in the left arm and loss of use of the hand, and presented a picture of a typical brachial plexus lesion. The friend disappeared 'back to work'. The patient said he did not want anyone to inform and worry his wife because she was in hospital, 50 miles away, expecting their first baby. To add authenticity to the story the friend telephoned later to say the wife had been delivered of twins.

So far he had not been given any drug and after being X-rayed he was admitted to the orthopedic ward. After a short while he complained of tightness in his chest and he 'coughed' up some blood which he proudly presented in his handkerchief. This made the staff suspicious because the sputum looked more like nasal mucus than that of a hemoptysis. He then began demanding a pain-killing injection. Very soon after this the nursing staff changed over, and the night superintendent recognized him and his elaborate story (including the twins) from a hospital she had worked in 6 months previously and 150 miles away! When the Rogues' Gallery was consulted it was found that a similar patient had used the identical presentation in at least three other widely scattered Accident and Emergency departments. Needless to say, when confronted he rapidly disappeared, dressing himself using both arms without difficulty.

Other unusual 'phoney' presentations encountered by the author include a locked knee with a history suggestive of a torn cartilage, acute sciatica, hemoptysis, and an 'axillary vein thrombosis' in which a tourniquet was later discovered tied round the upper arm.

MALINGERERS

Patients attending hospital with simulated symptoms or prolongation of disability after an injury, when they merely want to avoid returning to work or responsibility, are much harder to detect than the more dramatic hospital hoppers. Frequently the nursing staff first become suspicious. Malingerers are people of all sizes and ages; school children and elderly people are not exempt. The Accident and Emergency department is a chosen place for a malingerer to continue to attend as he may be treated by a different doctor every time he attends the department. It is, therefore, a sound practice to ensure that a returning patient should not attend for supervision more than three times without being reviewed by a more senior doctor, or referred back to his general practitioner who may know him better for his 'work-shy' or 'school-shy' behaviour.

Typical minor injuries which malingerers are prone to perpetuate are back injuries, chest injuries, with or without minor rib fractures, and wrist and ankle sprains. Wrist sprains are particularly common in teenage girls who are bored with their last few years at school, or whose parents are believed to 'misunderstand' them. Their phantom recurrent injuries subside when they leave school or get the attention they crave from a regular boyfriend.

Brought in dead (BID) or dead on arrival (DOA)

Patients involved in an accident or who collapse in the street, may die instantly or during transportation to hospital. The category 'brought in dead' or 'dead on arrival' poses some special problems for the staff in the Accident and Emergency department.

A few years ago these patients were never allowed entry into the department because of the difficulties that they presented to the staff. For example, the body became the responsibility of the department and the nursing staff had to check the patient's property, lay out the body, and thoroughly clean the trolley (gurney) and room before they could be used again. Consequently, receiving nurses were annoyed if the ambulance men brought in a patient they believed to be dead, because it disrupted the normal working of the department. Another consideration was the fact that little could be done if the patient appeared to be dead.

Nowadays the attitude has changed completely because of modern resuscitation methods and equipment and the ability to detect minimal signs of life by means of an ECG (EKG). There is also the fear that signs of life might be missed. This is a particularly sensitive matter especially in the eyes of the general public, particularly after cases of 'recovery' in the mortuary have appeared in the press or television.

In addition to these considerations the ritual cleansing of the admission room is no longer required so that the death of a patient in the Accident and Emergency department is less disruptive to the staff than in previous years.

It follows that except in cases where death is absolutely certain the doctor should not be expected to certify someone as dead in a small dark ambulance armed only with a stethoscope and an ophthalmoscope particularly if the patient is a young person or if the ambulance staff have been attempting resuscitation en route. Often the ambulance service will have sent a radio message to say they have a possible death and will indicate the expected time of their arrival, so that the nurse can alert the doctor, prepare the resuscitation room for the victim's reception and have the resuscitation and defibrillation equipment ready for use.

Two categories of patient demand particular care before they are abandoned as dead:

(1) Elderly people found collapsed at home in winter, either in or out of bed. They may be hypothermic (p. 258).
(2) Cases of apparent drowning (p. 96).

Patients in these groups not only look dead but may feel dead too!

Appendix

Adverse reactions to drugs

M. B. McILLMURRAY

Idiosyncratic reactions

These are unpredictable, unrelated to dose and previous exposure is not an essential feature. The most notable example is that which occurs with the phenothiazine group of drugs (including chlorpromazine, promazine, prochlorperazine, perphenazine and trifluoperazine). Curious abnormal movements of limbs, face and tongue occur, together with an irresistible urge to move about. As these drugs are frequently administered in the Accident and Emergency department, the nurse should be aware of these occasional frightening reactions. They are abolished by the anticholinergic drug, benztropine.

Hypersensitivity reactions

These are mediated by immunological mechanisms, and allergy sufferers are particularly prone to them. There are several types of hypersensitivity, but anaphylaxis, the immediate type, is the only one which concerns the Accident and Emergency nurse. Anaphylactic shock (p. 140) occurs when histamine and other substances are released from tissue stores as a result of the reaction between a drug and the patient's immune system. There is a sudden and catastrophic fall in blood pressure, pallor, sweating, cyanosis and vomiting. Breathlessness from bronchoconstriction occurs and death may follow. Treatment is urgent; 1 ml of adrenaline (epinephrine) injection BP (1 in 1000 solution) should be given intramuscularly to raise the blood pressure and dilate the airways. This may be followed by aminophylline 250 mg given by slow intravenous injection.

Anaphylaxis may follow the injection of a number of drugs, notably penicillin and antisera. Before any drug is given it is essential for the nurse to ask the patient about previous sensitivity reactions. Moreover, special care should be taken in patients with a history of asthma, infantile eczema or other allergic disorders. The nurse should consult the doctor before giving an injection if she is in any doubt. A solution of adrenaline 1 in 1000 and a sterile syringe should always be readily available.

When serum has to be given, as in suspected cases of tetanus (p. 24), the possibility of a reaction is greatly reduced if the following regime is observed. If there is no history of allergy, or of a previous injection of serum the required dose can be given. If serum has been given before, a test dose of 0.2 ml of serum should be given subcutaneously and the patient observed for 30 minutes. If there is no reaction, such as local erythema the remainder is given 30 minutes later. The patient is then observed for a further 30 minutes before he leaves the department.

Index